The laboratory investigation of liver disease

Leeds Poly

The laboratory investigation of liver disease

P. J. Johnson, MRCP
*Honorary Consultant Physician and Senior Lecturer,
Liver Unit, King's College Hospital School of Medicine,
London*

and

I. G. McFarlane, Ph.D., MRCPath.
*Consultant Biochemist and Hon. Senior Lecturer,
Liver Unit, King's College Hospital School of Medicine,
London*

Baillière Tindall

London Philadelphia Toronto Sydney Tokyo

Baillière Tindall
W. B. Saunders

24–28 Oval Road
London NW1 7DX, England

The Curtis Center
Independence Square West
Philadelphia, PA 19106-3399, USA

1 Goldthorne Avenue
Toronto, Ontario M8Z 5T9, Canada

Harcourt Brace Jovanovich Group (Australia) Pty Ltd
32–52 Smidmore Street
Marrickville, NSW 2204, Australia

Harcourt Brace Jovanovich Japan Inc.
Ichibancho Central Building, 22–1 Ichibancho
Chiyoda-ku, Tokyo 102, Japan

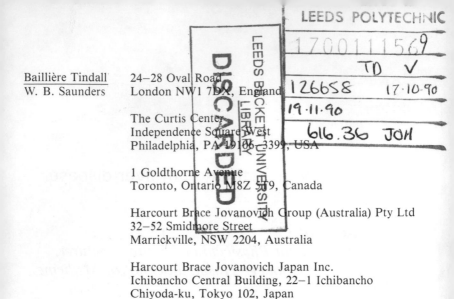

© 1989 Baillière Tindall

British Library Cataloguing in Publication Data

Is available

ISBN 0-7020-1376-5 ✓

Typeset by Mathematical Composition Setters Ltd, Salisbury
Printed in Great Britain by T J Press (Padstow) Ltd, Padstow, Cornwall.

Contents

To our wives, Susan and Barbara

Preface

Until about 30 years ago, the differential diagnosis of liver disease was fairly limited in scope. The clinician was mainly required to establish whether the disorder was acute or chronic and whether it was extrahepatic (in which case surgical intervention was the norm) or intrahepatic (when there was often little that could be offered to the patient other than bed rest and advice on diet). Developments in diagnostic techniques and treatment modalities, particularly during the past 10 to 15 years, present the clinician today with what can at times be a bewildering array of possible diagnoses and management options. Accurate diagnosis and monitoring of patients has become of paramount importance, because therapeutic intervention (including surgery) that may be appropriate in one liver disorder is often contraindicated in others, while delays in instituting therapy or failure to maintain adequate treatment in certain liver conditions can have disastrous consequences.

Several of the more sophisticated techniques that have been developed (e.g. ultrasonography, angiography, endoscopy, percutaneous liver biopsy) are quite costly and require highly trained personnel for their administration and interpretation and/or are invasive procedures that cannot be frequently repeated. Furthermore, the availability of many of these techniques is largely confined to specialist centres and, for initial diagnosis and subsequent follow-up of patients with liver disease, the majority of clinicians still have to rely on laboratory tests (on blood, urine and faecal specimens) performed by local laboratory services. However, here too there have been many developments and even experienced hepatologists and pathologists can sometimes find it difficult to grasp the complexities of interpretation of the numerous laboratory tests that have recently been evolved.

During several years of lecturing to medical and paramedical undergraduate and postgraduate students, we have been faced with a continuing problem in recommending suitable reference texts for the courses with which we have been involved. The information is available but it is scattered throughout a number of large (albeit excellent) tomes on clinical hepatology and in the medical and scientific journals. There seemed to be a need for a relatively small volume in which the essentials of the laboratory investigation of hepatic disorders could be drawn together for easy reference. Since none appeared to be forthcoming, we have undertaken the task ourselves.

This is not a technical manual. Rather, it is intended as an interpretative guide to the laboratory diagnosis and monitoring of liver disease. All of the widely available routine laboratory investigations are covered and many of the more specialized and newer tests have been included. In addition, we have tried to give as much background information as is possible within the constraints of the main aim of the book. We have anticipated that some may wish to read the book from cover to cover while others may use it more for quick reference on a day-to-day basis and, to accommodate both types of reader, some repetition of information has been unavoidable. We apologize to our more assiduous readers if they find this a little distracting.

The early chapters are arranged in groups of laboratory tests, while later chapters are more "disease-oriented" in the sense that they deal with the interpretation of results of the tests required for some of the more common difficult diagnostic problems that arise. We have deliberately excluded separate chapters on liver histology and bacteriology because these subjects are already more than adequately covered in reasonably condensed form in available specialist texts to which reference is made.

We hope that readers will find this book informative and, especially, that they will find it useful. Direct approaches with criticisms and suggestions for future editions will be most welcome.

Finally, we must express our gratitude to Drs G. J. M. Alexander, E. A. Fagan, W. L. Hutchison, W. Marshall, G. Mufti, J. M. Tredger and D. Vergani for reading early drafts of the various chapters and for their many helpful suggestions, and to Dr Roger Williams for his continuing and unwavering support over many years.

1

An introduction to liver disease

1.1 Introduction

This chapter is intended to present a brief and simplified outline of the causes, classification and consequences of the more common types of liver disease for those readers whose background is not in the practice of clinical medicine. It also provides a summary of the classification of liver disease that is used in this text.

Liver disease is most readily classified according to its aetiology (Table 1.1). The "stage" of the disease process (acute, subacute, or chronic) and the pathological state of the liver (as defined histologically, or assessed clinically) is often added to form a diagnosis. For example, rather than simply stating that a patient has alcoholic liver disease, a diagnosis of acute alcoholic hepatitis or alcoholic cirrhosis imparts more precise information. Furthermore, the signs, symptoms and management problems often relate more closely to the liver pathology than its aetiology. Since the liver has only a limited number of responses to the various pathological insults, it is

TABLE 1.1. Classification of liver disease according to aetiology

Viral	*Toxic/drug induced*	*Autoimmune*
Hepatitis A	Alcohol	Chronic active hepatitis
Hepatitis B	Drugs	Primary biliary cirrhosis
Hepatitis non-A, non-B	Poisons	
Epstein–Barr		
Cytomegalovirus		
Metabolic	*Biliary-tract obstruction*	*Vascular*
Haemochromatosis	Tumours	Budd Chiari syndrome
Wilson's disease	Strictures	Portal vein thrombosis
The hereditary	Gallstones	Veno-occlusive disease
hyperbilirubinaemias	Sclerosing cholangitis	
	Biliary atresia	
Bacterial	*Cryptogenic*	*Neoplastic*
Tuberculosis		Primary (Table 1.7)
Pyogenic-liver abscess		Secondary
Protozoal	*Miscellaneous*	*Helminthic*
Kala-azar	Polycystic liver disease	Ascariasis
Amoebiasis	Congenital hepatic	Toxocariasis
Malaria	fibrosis	Chlonorchis
		Schistosomiasis

simpler to consider the clinical picture associated with these responses rather than all the different aetiologies individually. Thus patients with cirrhosis suffer much the same range of problems irrespective of whether the cirrhosis is attributable to excessive alcohol consumption or some form of chronic viral hepatitis.

1.2 Acute hepatitis and its sequelae [1]

Acute inflammation of the liver, associated with hepatocyte damage or death, can be caused by viruses or toxins (under which heading we include drugs and alcohol) though the mechanisms of cell damage differ widely. Symptoms vary depending on the severity of the process

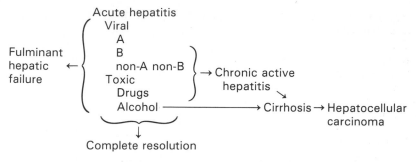

FIG. 1.1. Possible sequelae of acute hepatitis. Alcohol is not usually regarded as a cause of fulminant hepatic failure, but the picture of severe alcoholic hepatitis is very similar and the prognosis equally grave.

and range from none to jaundice and lethargy. There are three main possible outcomes: (i) complete resolution; (ii) progression to chronic liver disease, particularly chronic active hepatitis, and (iii) acute liver failure (ALF) (Fig 1.1). ALF implies the development of severe hepatic dysfunction within 6 months of the first symptoms and in the absence of any pre-existing liver disease. The characteristic clinical feature is encephalopathy usually associated with severe coagulopathy, and when these features develop very quickly (within 8 weeks) after the first symptoms the condition is known as fulminant hepatic failure (FHF)—a rare but often fatal complication of acute liver disease [2].

1.3 Chronic liver disease and the concept of cirrhosis [3,4]

The term chronic here implies that the disease will neither cause death during the acute illness, nor resolve spontaneously. In the case of acute viral hepatitis the chronic stage is said to have been reached when signs (clinical or biochemical) and/or symptoms of liver disease have been present for more than 6 months [5]. Chronic hepatitis may be sub-divided on histological grounds into *chronic active hepatitis* (CAH) and *chronic persistent hepatitis*. The former is more likely to progress to liver failure and cirrhosis; the latter is usually benign, but may occasionally progress to CAH.

Cirrhosis is not a clinical diagnosis but a pathological description of the liver when there is diffuse hepatic fibrosis, nodular regeneration and disturbance of the normal hepatic architecture, i.e. distortion of the relation of the portal tracts to the central veins. It is the irreversible end-result of any chronic process which leads to recurrent waves of cell death and attempts by the liver at regeneration. A "precirrhotic" stage in which there is extensive fibrosis but no definite nodule formation is often recognized.

Other than hepatitis A (infectious hepatitis), any of the conditions described in Section 1.2 may lead via chronic liver disease to cirrhosis. There are, in addition, a number of other conditions which do not usually have an acute presentation but which may also lead to cirrhosis — including autoimmune chronic active hepatitis, primary biliary cirrhosis and haemochromatosis (Table 1.2). These conditions and those mentioned in Section 1.2 may progress to cirrhosis without producing any symptoms. Likewise, cirrhosis does not always cause symptoms, in which case it is said to be "well compensated", i.e. although the liver is damaged there is sufficient reserve to carry out its normal functions. When the cirrhosis becomes "decompensated" the symptoms attributable to the combination of portal hypertension and liver failure may supervene (Table 1.3). The severity of cirrhosis can also be described by the use of Child's classification or Pugh's modification thereof (Table 1.4), [6].

1.3.1 Portal hypertension

Blood draining from the intra-abdominal part of the alimentary tract, pancreas, spleen and gall-bladder reaches the liver via the portal vein which forms the first part of the dual blood supply of the liver, the second part coming from the hepatic artery. Many liver diseases (Table 1.5), particularly cirrhosis, cause an increased resistance to blood flow through the portal vein and a consequent increase in the portal venous pressure. This, in turn, leads to the development of collateral channels between the portal and lower pressure systemic circulation. Such channels are seen as varicose veins in the submucosa of the oesophagus, stomach and rectum, and on the anterior abdominal wall.

The clinical importance of portal hypertension is two-fold. First, there may be catastrophic haemorrhage from the oesophageal or gastric varices, and second, the natural filtering and detoxifying functions of the liver are bypassed and gut-derived antigens, bacteria, drugs and gut hormones may enter the systemic circulation — the consequences of so-called "portal-systemic shunting". Of particular importance is the failure of the liver to detoxify nitrogenous compounds (such as ammonia) produced by the action of gut bacteria on dietary protein. This is the mechanism of portal-systemic

TABLE 1.2. Causes of cirrhosis, according to aetiology. The commoner types are in bold letters: overall, alcohol is responsible for most cases in the West and viral hepatitis for most cases in the rest of the world.

Alcohol
Hepatitis B, non-A, non-B
Autoimmune chronic active hepatitis
Primary biliary cirrhosis
Cryptogenic cirrhosis

Haemochromatosis
Secondary biliary cirrhosis
Wilson's disease
Neonatal hepatitis
Alpha-1 antitrypsin deficiency and other genetic disorders

TABLE 1.3. Signs and symptoms of portal hypertension and liver failure

Complication of cirrhosis	Possible clinical consequences
Oesophageal varices	Variceal haemorrhage
Portal-systemic encephalopathy	Subtle changes in mood to deep coma
Ascites and peripheral oedema	Cosmetic changes, discomfort when extreme
Hormonal disturbances	Impotence, infertility, glucose intolerance
Splenomegaly	Hypersplenism (low platelet and white cell counts)
Hyperbilirubinaemia	Jaundice

The "cutaneous stigmata of chronic liver disease"
    Arterial spiders (often inaccurately called "spider naevi")
    Liver palms
    White nails (leuconychia)

Depending on the nature of the disease and its stage, different physiological functions of the liver fail at different times so that not all the consequences listed above occur at the same time in a particular patient. The "cutaneous signs" are useful in clinical diagnosis but do not cause symptoms. The extent to which liver failure and portal hypertension are individually responsible for these signs and symptoms is, in most instances, controversial and difficult to ascertain. It is probably safe to assume that in most cases both are involved.

TABLE 1.4. Child's classification (modified by Pugh) for assessing severity of liver disease. Patients scoring 5 or 6 points ("Grade A") are considered a good operative risk, those scoring 7 to 9 points a moderate operative risk, and those with between 10 and 15 points a poor operative risk. Encephalopathy is grade 1–4, 1 being mild confusion, 4 being coma. The system was initially devised to assess hepatic reserve in patients requiring surgery, particularly portocaval shunting for variceal haemorrhage.

Clinical and Biochemical Measurements	Points scored for increasing abnormalities		
	1	2	3
Ascites	Absent	Slight	Moderate
Encephalopathy (Grade)	None	1 and 2	3 and 4
Bilirubin (umol/l)	<25	25–40	>40
Albumin (g/l)	>35	28–35	<28
Prothrombin time (seconds longer than control)	1–4	4–6	>6

TABLE 1.5. Some causes of portal hypertension in relation to the site of resistance.

Prehepatic
Portal or splenic vein thrombosis
Tropical splenomegaly[a]

Intrahepatic
Cirrhosis of any type
Precirrhotic chronic liver disease
Drugs and toxins: azathioprine (high dose), vinyl chloride monomer, arsenic
Idiopathic[a]
Congenital hepatic fibrosis

Suprahepatic
Constrictive pericarditis
Right ventricular failure
Budd–Chiari syndrome (hepatic vein thrombosis)

[a]Portal pressure is a function of blood flow as well as resistance. Increased flow is sometimes implicated in the development of portal hypertension.

encephalopathy, a complication of portal hypertension and chronic liver disease which may lead to psychological disturbances and ultimately coma. Portal-systemic shunts may also be created surgically to decrease portal pressure and thereby treat, or decrease the likelihood of, variceal haemorrhage.

1.4 Cholestasis

Failure of bile secretion ("intrahepatic cholestasis") or bile flow ("extrahepatic cholestasis") is a frequent clinical problem with many possible causes (Table 1.6). Extrahepatic cholestasis (also known as "obstruction") may not be, strictly speaking, always due to liver disease because the obstruction may occur anywhere between the hepatic ducts and the sphincter of Oddi (Fig 1.2). Whatever the cause of cholestasis, the initial symptom is often itching (pruritus) followed by jaundice together with dark urine (due to conjugated bilirubin) and pale stools (due to failure of bile pigments to reach the gut). Typical additional clinical findings in the case of *extrahepatic* obstruction are abdominal pain, a palpable gall-bladder or other abdominal mass,

TABLE 1.6. Some causes of intra- and extra-hepatic cholestasis: several other conditions including acute alcoholic and viral hepatitis may pass through a cholestatic phase.

Intrahepatic cholestasis	Extrahepatic cholestasis	
Mechanical		
Biliary atresia	Gallstones	
Primary biliary cirrhosis	Strictures	(post-operative or
Sclerosing cholangitis		inflammatory)
Metastatic tumour	Tumours	(of bile ducts or pancreas)
Non-mechanical		
Drugs		
Septicaemia		
Parenteral nutrition		
Lymphomas		
Oestrogens and pregnancy		

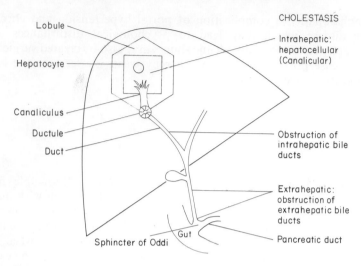

FIG. 1.2. Types of cholestasis (from Erlinger) (see Suggested further reading).

evidence of cholangitis and a history of previous biliary tract surgery. Unrelieved, and depending on the degree of obstruction, these may lead to death or occasionally, secondary biliary cirrhosis.

Biliary cirrhosis is due to long-term, usually partial, biliary obstruction and has characteristic histological features. In *primary* biliary cirrhosis (PBC) the cause of the obstruction is not known and, confusingly, true cirrhosis as already defined (Section 1.3), only develops late in the course of the disease.

1.5 Neoplastic disease of the liver

Primary neoplasms of the liver may arise from malignant transformation of any of the normal hepatic cells (Table 1.7). The benign tumours are very rare, and of these only the adenoma is of any clinical importance, being occasionally associated with long-term oral-contraceptive use. The malignant tumours all typically present with the triad of upper abdominal pain (usually sited in the right upper quadrant), weight loss and hepatomegaly and lead to death within

TABLE 1.7. Benign and malignant tumours of the liver according to cell of origin

Cell	Tumour	
	Benign	Malignant
Hepatocyte	Hepatic adenoma	Hepatocellular carcinoma
		Hepatoblastoma[a]
Bile duct	Cholangioma	Cholangiocarcinoma
Endothelial	Haemangioma	Angiosarcoma

[a] Hepatoblastoma is a tumour of childhood.

two years of diagnosis either as a result of liver failure (Section 1.3) or cancer cachexia. Hepatocellular carcinoma is by far the commonest of the three primary tumours and usually arises as a complication of long-standing cirrhosis (Section 1.3 and Fig. 1.1). The liver is the commonest site of metastatic (secondary) deposits. Although symptoms are similar to those of primary liver tumours, they are often overshadowed by symptoms from the primary tumour or metastatic disease at other sites.

The term *hepatoma* is sometimes used instead of primary liver cancer (i.e. any of the primary liver cancers) or, more often, specifically for hepatocellular carcinoma.

References

1. Vyas GN, *et al.* Viral Hepatitis and Liver Disease. New York: Grune & Stratton, 1984.
2. Trey C and Davidson CS. In: Progress in Liver Disease, Vol III (Popper H, Schaffner F, Eds). New York: Grune & Stratton, 1970: 282–298.
3. Anthony PP, *et al.* Bull WHO 1978; 55: 521–540.
4. Leevy CM and Tygstrup N (Eds). Standardisation of Nomenclature, Diagnostic Criteria, and Diagnostic Methodology for Diseases of the Liver and Biliary Tract. Basel: S. Karger, 1976:
5. De Groote J, *et al.* Lancet 1968; ii; 626–628.
6. Pugh RNH, *et al.* Br J Surg 1973; 60: 646–649.

Suggested further reading

Erlinger S. What is cholestasis in 1985? J Hepatol, 1985; **1** 687–693.

Galambos JT. Cirrhosis. Philadelphia: WB Saunders, 1979.

Johnson PJ and Williams R (Eds). Liver Tumours. Baillière's Clinical Gastroenterology 1987; Vol. 1, No. 1.

Sherlock S. Diseases of the Liver and Biliary System. Oxford: Blackwell Scientific, 1987.

2

The standard liver function tests

2.1 Introduction

As Sherlock has pointed out "the multiple functions of the liver are only exceeded by the number of biochemical methods designed to test them" [1]. The original aim of such tests was to answer two questions. In a particular patient, is liver disease present and, if so, what is the nature and severity of the disease?

The first question is pertinent in situations where there is no clinical evidence of liver disease, for example during the incubation period of viral hepatitis or during therapy with a drug known to be potentially hepatotoxic. The second is clearly important before treatment is started, or a prognosis given. A prerequisite of therapy is a precise diagnosis and the vast increase in the number of diagnostic modalities (immunological, virological and imaging) reflects this and testifies to the inadequacy of the standard so-called "liver function tests

(LFTs)"[*] in this area. It should be recognized from the outset, therefore, that these tests offer little quantitative information (i.e. the extent of liver damage) and measure dysfunction rather than function and survive from the days of limited diagnostic and therapeutic options. Nonetheless, the vast experience that has accrued with these tests, their simplicity, the ease with which results can be stored, and the fact that they are observer-independent all keep LFTs in demand. For this reason, and because of the new-found role in monitoring therapy, the LFTs remain the first line of investigation, and an important part of the day-to-day management of patients with liver disease. It is, however, important to be aware of the limitations of their use because *over interpretation is frequent and may lead to serious mismanagement.*

The "standard" LFTs are usually considered to include the following three groups:

(i) serum bilirubin concentration — sometimes included are separate estimations of the conjugated and unconjugated fractions, and urinary urobilinogen and bilirubin;

(ii) serum enzyme activities — commonly used are the aminotransferases, alkaline phosphatase, and gamma-glutamyl transpeptidase or 5'-nucleotidase;

(iii) plasma proteins — total protein, albumin and, by subtraction, serum globulin levels.

Several workers have sought to improve on this battery of tests and gain a genuine measurement of liver function, i.e. a quantitative assessment of functional hepatic mass. From such efforts were derived "second-generation" LFTs based on the capacity of the liver to clear exogenous compounds such as bromsulphthalein, indocyanine green, aminopyrine or caffeine, or endogenous compounds such as bile acids (Chapter 3).

In this chapter we consider first the physiological and biochemical basis of each test, laying particular emphasis on those aspects which are clinically important, then their use in clinical practice, and finally patterns of abnormality within the whole battery of LFTs as seen in specific conditions.

---

[*] Some authorities prefer to designate these tests simply as "liver tests" to emphasize that no claim is made to assess function.

2.2   Bilirubin and bile pigment metabolism [2]

Accurate interpretation of the clinical signs and the laboratory tests involved in the differential diagnosis of the jaundiced patient requires an understanding of the physiology of bile pigments.

2.2.1   Formation of bilirubin

Bilirubin is an orange–yellow pigment derived from haem (Fe-protoporphyrin IX). Metabolic studies using radiolabelled precursors of bilirubin show that there are two peaks of production. The first, between 0 and 2 days after the administration of the isotope, represents breakdown of haem containing hepatic proteins such as catalase, myoglobin and the cytochromes and accounts for 20% of bilirubin production. The second peak at 120 days is attributable to the destruction of effete red blood cells; this represents the major source of haem and, ultimately, bilirubin. A small fraction of the "early labelled" bilirubin is due to ineffective erythropoiesis, and this may become a significant source of bilirubin in conditions such as pernicious anaemia and thalassaemia.

The initial and rate-limiting step in the production of bilirubin is oxidation of haem to biliverdin (a green pigment) followed by reduction to bilirubin, with the production of an equimolar amount of carbon monoxide and ferric iron. About $500\,\mu$mol (275 mg) of bilirubin is produced each day (Fig. 2.1). These reactions occur in the reticuloendothelial system, predominantly in the liver, spleen and bone marrow. The "free" or "unconjugated" bilirubin so produced binds tightly, but reversibly, to albumin ($K_a = 10^{-9}$) in a molar ratio of 1 : 1 at normal concentrations, but additional binding sites of lower affinity are recruited in hyperbilirubinaemic states.

2.2.2   Transport

This unconjugated bilirubin is insoluble in water at physiological pH because of intramolecular hydrogen bonds which prevent ionization of the two terminal carboxylic acid groupings (Fig. 2.2). Binding to albumin stops extrahepatic (particularly brain) uptake of the lipid-soluble, potentially toxic, unconjugated bilirubin and permits transport to the liver. Albumin is capable of binding up to $400\,\mu$mol$\,$l^{-1} but

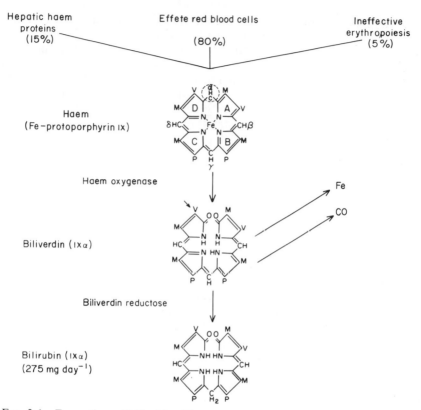

FIG. 2.1 Formation of bilirubin. The rate-limiting enzyme haem oxygenase opens the α-methene bridge of the haem molecule.

other anions such as thyroxine and some drugs can compete for the albumin binding sites and, thereby, displace bilirubin (see Section 2.11.3). (A third bilirubin fraction "firmly (?covalently) bound" to albumin exists in the serum of patients with long-standing cholestasis [3, 4]; this is of clinical but not physiological significance (see Section 2.11.2).)

2.2.3 Uptake and conjugation

Following dissociation of the albumin–bilirubin complex, bilirubin enters the hepatocyte across the sinusoidal membrane by a carrier-mediated process where it binds to cytosolic proteins, mainly ligandin (glutathione S transferase B). The transfer is bidirectional and this presumably accounts for the small amount (< 1%) of conjugated bilirubin that can be detected in normal serum. Bilirubin is conjugated in the endoplasmic reticulum with glucuronic acid (by the enzyme uridine diphosphoglucuronate glucoronyl transferase) to form mono- and di-glucuronides, thus rendering it water soluble and available for biliary excretion (Fig. 2.2).

2.2.4 Excretion and enterohepatic circulation (Fig. 2.3)

The bilirubin conjugates (mainly diglucuronides) are excreted in the bile, probably by an energy-dependent, carrier-mediated process,

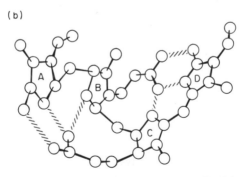

FIG. 2.2 (a) The unfolded structure of bilirubin showing the site of glucuronic acid conjugation which breaks the hydrogen bonding and results in the molecule becoming water soluble. (b) The folded structure showing the extensive internal hydrogen bonding. (From Schmid [2], with permission.)

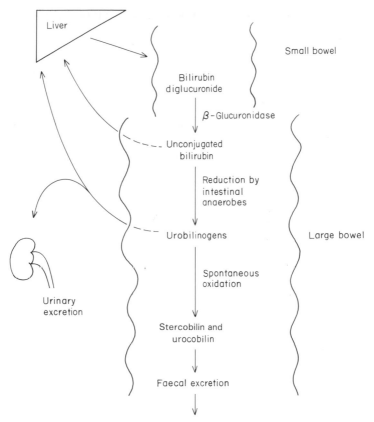

FIG. 2.3 The enterohepatic circulation of bilirubin and urobilinogen.

because it occurs against a significant concentration gradient. Some conjugates will be deconjugated by glucuronidases (from the small bowel and of bacterial origin) and, being lipid soluble, will be reabsorbed into the hepatic portal system and ultimately be reconjugated and re-excreted. Bile pigments reaching the colon undergo bacterial degradation to urobilinogen and stercobilinogen. About 20% of this group of compounds also undergoes an enterohepatic circulation (a small fraction, 2–5%, reaches the systemic circulation and is excreted by the kidney). The remainder is excreted in the faeces. Some urobilinogens oxidize spontaneously to stercobilin, an orange–brown pigment responsible for stool colour. Normal serum bilirubin, being unconjugated and thus water insoluble, is not excreted by the kidney and is not detectable in the urine.

2.3 Diagnosis and significance of hyperbilirubinaemia

In more than 95% of the apparently normal adult population, the serum bilirubin concentration is below $25\,\mu mol\,l^{-1}$ [5] and this can be considered the upper limit of the reference range (Fig. 2.4). Above $50\,\mu mol\,l^{-1}$ bilirubin, hyperbilirubinaemia can often be detected as jaundice by experienced observers, and when in excess of $100\,\mu mol\,l^{-1}$ patients' relatives will usually pass comment. The level of bilirubin in the serum of an individual is determined by the balance between production and clearance. Although less than 500 mg of bilirubin is produced each day, the normal liver is capable of conjugating up to

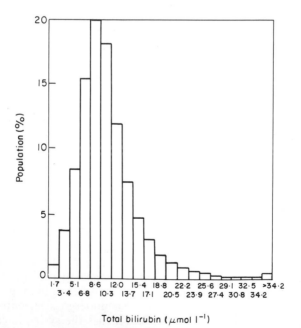

FIG. 2.4 Distribution of serum bilirubin concentration in 18 454 healthy men. (From Bailey *et al.* [5] with permission.)

$1500 \, \text{mg day}^{-1}$. This large functional reserve is one reason why the serum bilirubin is an insensitive test for liver disease.

The absolute level of serum bilirubin is of little help in establishing a diagnosis. Quantification is, however, important in monitoring the progress of disease such as primary biliary cirrhosis, where changes are of prognostic significance (see Section 2.13), neonatal hepatitis (Section 2.11.4), assessing response to treatment (such as surgical relief of bile-duct obstruction), or to detect hyperbilirubinaemia that is suspected but not clinically apparent. In addition, the absolute level of bilirubin is important in prescribing the correct dose of certain cytotoxic agents. For example, in patients with malignant liver disease treated with doxorubicin (adriamycin), the dose must be decreased in the presence of hyperbilirubinaemia to avoid undue myelosuppression. The highest concentrations of bilirubin (sometimes approaching $1000 \, \mu \text{mol l}^{-1}$) are seen when conjugated jaundice of any cause is complicated by renal failure (see Chapter 3).

2.3.1 Basis of tests for quantification of bilirubin and its conjugated and unconjugated fractions

Conjugated bilirubin is reacted with diazotized sulphanilic acid to produce an azobilirubin, a coloured compound which can be quantitated easily. This fraction has been termed "direct reacting", implying that the reaction takes place in the absence of alcohol. If alcohol (or caffeine) is added before the reaction takes place, the intramolecular hydrogen bonds of the unconjugated fraction are broken (Section 2.2.2) and total bilirubin can be measured. The unconjugated, or "indirect reacting" bilirubin, (i.e. that fraction which only reacts after addition of alcohol) is estimated as the difference between the two. Thus,

Diazo reaction + alcohol   *Diazo reaction, no alcohol*

Total bilirubin   —   Conjugated bilirubin   =   Unconjugated bilirubin
(direct reacting)   (indirect reacting)

While there is no doubt that this method is of great clinical value, its limitations should be recognized. At levels of serum bilirubin below $50 \, \mu \text{mol l}^{-1}$ the test does not permit accurate measurement of the two major fractions. Recently, a new procedure involving alkaline methanolysis and high-performance liquid chromatography (AM-HPLC) has shown convincingly that there is, in fact, not a precise relationship between "indirect" and "unconjugated" and "direct" and "conjugated" bilirubins, respectively: direct reacting levels overestimate conjugated bilirubin at low concentrations and underestimate it at high levels. Techniques permitting accurate estimations of the two fractions at low total bilirubin concentrations may soon become available routinely and preliminary evidence suggests that estimation of conjugated bilirubin may be a very specific and sensitive test of hepatobiliary dysfunction [6]. At present, however, the main indication for distinguishing the two fractions of bilirubin lies in the diagnosis of haemolytic jaundice and certain of the congenital hyperbilirubinaemias.

2.3.2 Urinary bilirubin and urobilinogen

Urinary bilirubin can be reliably detected by the use of commercially available dipsticks. A positive test indicates hepatic or biliary tract dysfunction and, as noted above, bilirubinuria may be present before the bilirubin level starts to rise in the blood. The test remains an invaluable screening test in general practice, although it is less used in hospitals where there is usually ready access to serum estimations. Accurate measurement of urinary urobilinogen concentrations is more difficult. If bile pigments reach the gut in reduced amounts (as in obstructive jaundice) then the amount of urobilinogen in the urine will be decreased accordingly. If no urobilinogen can be detected on repeated testing over several days, complete biliary-tract obstruction, the most common cause of which is malignant disease such as pancreatic carcinoma, may be assumed. However, there are now much more reliable ways of diagnosing malignant obstruction (such as ultrasonography) and urinary urobilinogen is becoming an obsolete test.

2.4 Haemolytic jaundice

As already noted, the normal bilirubin level is determined by the balance between bilirubin production and clearance. The production rate is directly related to the red-cell survival time and, as this becomes shorter in haemolytic disorders, so the bilirubin level rises in direct proportion. The maximum compensatory increase in red-cell production that the bone marrow can achieve is about eight-fold and this corresponds with a serum bilirubin of not more than $75\,\mu\mathrm{mol\,l^{-1}}$. Thus the common chronic haemolytic disorders present with mild unconjugated hyperbilirubinaemia with no bilirubin in the urine; hence the alternative term for haemolytic jaundice — "acholuric jaundice". Serum aminotransferase activity may be slightly elevated (of red cell rather than liver origin), and an increased reticulocyte count is also characteristic. Urinary and faecal urobilinogen levels will be increased, but these changes also occur in hepatocellular jaundice and are, therefore, of no diagnostic value.

There are two situations in which serum bilirubin levels of more than $75\,\mu\mathrm{mol\,l^{-1}}$ may occur in haemolytic anaemia. First, when there is associated liver damage and the clearance is compromised (and an increasing fraction of the bilirubin will therefore be conjugated). Examples of this are seen in Wilson's disease and acute alcoholic hepatitis where a severe haemolytic jaundice may be the presenting feature (Zieve's syndrome, see Chapter 4). Secondly, in acute haemolytic crises (in sickle-cell anaemia, for example), the production rate will exceed the maximum rate of hepatic clearance — the bilirubin will again be increasingly conjugated, and the haemoglobin level will fall because red cells are destroyed faster than they can be replaced by the marrow. It is in complicated situations such as these that distinction between conjugated and unconjugated bilirubin may be most useful diagnostically.

2.5 The congenital hyperbilirubinaemias [7] (Table 2.1)

The congenital hyperbilirubinaemias are considered here because their main interest to the general reader is in illustrating specific disturbances in the metabolism of bile pigments. Apart from Gilbert's syndrome these conditions are rare and, generally speaking, the other liver-function tests are normal. The more common types of jaundice are, by contrast, associated with other liver function test abnormalities and are, therefore, considered later, after the discussion of the remaining LFTs. The congenital hyperbilirubinaemias are conventionally separated into conjugated and unconjugated types, *the latter being defined as occurring when less than 20% of an elevated bilirubin level is in the conjugated state.*

TABLE 2.1 Differential diagnosis of the congenital hyperbilirubinaemias

	Gilbert's syndrome	Crigler–Najjar Syndrome		Dubin–Johnson syndrome	Rotor's syndrome
		Type 1	Type 2		
Incidence	Common	Rare	Rare	Uncommon	Rare
Mode of inheritance	(?) Autosomal dominant	Autosomal recessive	Unknown	Autosomal recessive	Autosomal recessive
Clinical features other than jaundice	None	Kernicterus; deep jaundice and death in early infancy	Usually None	None	None
Serum bilirubin (μmol l^{-1})	Variable Normal to 100	300–600	100–400	Variable 35–100	35–100
Other LFTs	Normal	Normal	Normal	Normal	Normal
BSP clearance	Reduced	Normal	Normal	Reduced with secondary rise at 100 min	Reduced: no secondary rise
Age of onset	Any, usually adolescence	Within first two days of life	Within first year of life	Early adult life. Often revealed in contraceptive-pill. Pregnancy	Childhood
Phenobarbitone lowers serum bilirubin	Yes	No	Yes	Yes	Yes

2.5.1 Unconjugated types

The *Crigler–Najjar* syndrome is an extremely rare condition, inherited in an autosomal recessive manner and caused by a deficiency of UDP-glucuronyl transferase. The syndrome presents in the first 48 h of life with jaundice which rapidly increases to between 20 and 40 times the upper limit of the serum bilirubin reference range. In the absence of treatment, kernicterus develops, and death ensues within the first year of life. A second, less severe type (type 2) is also recognized in which the bilirubin level is less than 20 times the upper limit of the reference range, the jaundice may occur later in life, and neurological damage is less severe.

By contrast, *Gilbert's syndrome* is an entirely benign condition which causes asymptomatic episodes of mild jaundice (up to five times

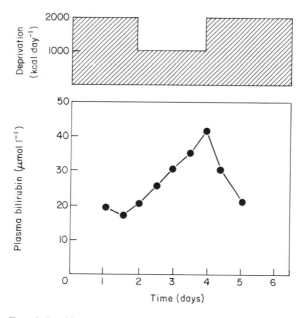

FIG. 2.5 Changes in serum bilirubin in response to caloric deprivation. Serum bilirubin rises in normal subjects in response to starvation, but the rise is much more pronounced in those with Gilbert's syndrome in whom the phenomenon can be used as a diagnostic test.

the upper limit of the reference range), which may be occasioned by intercurrent illnesses or caloric deprivation. Results of other LFTs are normal, as is the hepatic architecture. The importance of the condition lies in its recognition so that the patient is spared intensive investigation.

It is considered by some that Gilbert's syndrome represents one end of the normal distribution of serum bilirubin (see Section 2.3.2 and Fig. 2.4) and the observation that there seem to be several different underlying mechanisms involved does not rule out this possibility. Decreased hepatic bilirubin uptake is the commonest mechanism, but decreased bilirubin conjugation (reduced hepatic UDP glucuronyl transferase activity) is demonstrable in some. Following an intravenous dose of 500 mg of nicotinic acid, there is a two- to three-fold increase in plasma unconjugated bilirubin over the next 3 h. In normal subjects, or those with haemolytic jaundice, the level does not double. The test is not widely used because its specificity has been called into question and the nicotinic acid makes patients feel ill. Similar changes are seen after caloric restriction and this too has been used as a diagnostic test (Fig. 2.5). A decrease in the ratio of conjugated to total bilirubin (estimated by AM-HPLC (see Section 2.3.1) may be the most characteristic abnormality) [6].

It is important to emphasize the relative frequency of these two congenital abnormalities. Patients with the Crigler–Najjar syndrome will be seen once or twice in the lifetime of most paediatricians and most other physicians will never see a single case; by contrast, Gilbert's syndrome is a common occurrence in clinical practice, affecting perhaps 1% of the normal population.

2.5.2 Conjugated types

The *Dubin–Johnson syndrome* is a mild, largely asymptomatic, chronic intermittent jaundice due to a defect of hepatic excretion of conjugated bilirubin and other organic anions. Presentation is usually in early adult life and in women the first clinical attack of jaundice is often precipitated by the use of oral contraceptive preparations. Characteristically the gall-bladder fails to opacify on oral cholecystography. The diagnosis is usually easy to make because the liver biopsy appears black due to an unidentified pigment and the bromsulphthalein (BSP) (Chapter 3) test shows a secondary rise at about 100 min due to reflux of the conjugated BSP (Chapter 3).

An abnormal ratio of urinary coproporphyrin I : III has also been described. In normal subjects about 75% is in the isomer III form, whereas in patients with Dubin–Johnson syndrome 90% is in the I form, probably as a result of defective biliary excretion of coproporphyrinogen III.

The clinical features of *Rotor's syndrome* are similar to those of the Dubin–Johnson syndrome but the former may be distinguished by the lack of pigmentation in the liver biopsy, normal patterns of porphyrin excretion and the absence of a secondary rise in BSP test. The underlying mechanism appears to be defective uptake and/or storage of organic anions.

2.6 Serum enzyme activities

2.6.1 Alkaline phosphatase

2.6.1.1 Physiology and biochemistry

The term alkaline phosphatase (ALP) is used to describe a group of enzymes which hydrolyse phosphate esters at alkaline pH. ALP is present in several tissues, but the serum enzyme activity mainly comprises contributions from liver, bone, intestine and, during pregnancy, the placenta. The liver-derived isoenzyme is located on the exterior surface of the bile canalicular membrane and probably enters the bloodstream via the paracellular pathway (i.e. regurgitation from the canaliculus via the intracellular junction complex (Section 2.11.3) and directly across the plasma membrane). ALP may play a role in transport of bile acids into bile.

2.6.1.2 Basis of the clinical test

Activities of biliary and serum ALP rise in the face of bile duct obstruction and this forms the basis of its clinical usefulness. The elevation is due neither to failure of the liver to clear serum ALP (as would be the case for bilirubin) nor to the release of ALP from damaged hepatocytes (as in the case of the aminotransferases). Rather, several pieces of evidence suggest that bile-duct obstruction stimulates hepatic synthesis of alkaline phosphatase.

In rats the increased serum activity which follows bile-duct obstruction is due to increased translation of the mRNA, not increased transcription. The increased activity can be shown to be of biliary origin and no rise in serum ALP occurs if protein and RNA synthesis are blocked. However, mechanisms other than induction of hepatic ALP synthesis are also important. For example, only if elevated levels of bile acids are present are high levels of hepatic ALP reflected in the serum. Some evidence suggests that there is a cytosolic form of alkaline phosphatase as well as the membrane-bound enzyme [8].

2.6.1.3 Use in clinical practice

Any obstruction to the bile duct may lead to an increase in ALP activity. The obstruction may be at any level from high in the intrahepatic ducts (as in primary biliary cirrhosis or space-occupying lesions including granulomas) down to common bile duct (due to gallstones, bile-duct strictures or tumour). The rise in ALP may precede the onset of jaundice and, in those situations where surgical relief is possible, the return of serum bilirubin to the normal range often precedes that of ALP. A particularly characteristic picture is of elevated ALP activity in the presence of normal serum bilirubin concentration and this is highly suspicious of a space-occupying lesion, particularly intrahepatic tumour which, presumably, causes local biliary obstruction.

2.6.1.4 Overcoming the lack of tissue specificity

Increases in serum ALP activity are not unique to liver disease. They occur in pregnancy, during periods of rapid bone growth in childhood and adolescence, and as a consequence of pathology at extrahepatic sites (bone disease and certain malignant tumours), but they can be misinterpreted as evidence of liver disease.

This problem can be overcome by performing starch or poly-acrylamide-gel electrophoresis on the serum sample and staining the gels specifically for ALP. Normally, three distinct bands will be seen on the gels: corresponding to the liver, bone and intestinal ALP isoenzymes (Chapter 8). Additional bands are usually seen in pregnancy (the placental AP isoenzyme) and in patients with malignant liver disease (Chapter 8). The technique is only semiquantitative but it is nearly always visually obvious to which of the isoenzymes the increase in total ALP activity is due.

An alternative approach is to repeat the standard ALP assay after first heating the serum sample at $56\,^{\circ}$C for 15 min. The liver and bone isoenzymes are sensitive to this treatment and, if the increased total ALP activity is due to either of these, it will be reduced to about 40% and 15%, respectively, of the original value. The placental isoenzyme remains unaffected and, if this is the cause of the elevated ALP, the activity will remain the same after heat treatment. Obviously, this method is not as discriminatory as the electrophoretic separation of the isoenzymes, but it is easier to perform and can be used as a rough guide.

In practice, however, when there is doubt about the source of the increased ALP it is customary to examine the results in relation to any changes in other enzymes, elevation in the activities of which are more liver specific. Thus, if the gamma-glutamyl transpeptidase (GGTP), leucine aminopeptidase (LAP) or the 5′-nucleotidase (5′-NT) are also elevated, it may be inferred that the increased ALP is probably of liver origin (Section 2.7.1).

2.6.2 The aminotransferases

2.6.2.1 Physiology and biochemistry

These enzymes, previously designated (and still frequently referred to) as "transaminases", catalyse the transfer of an amino group from an α-amino acid to an α-keto acid. The two most widely measured for clinical purposes are aspartate aminotransferase (AST) [previously known as glutamic oxaloacetic transaminase (GOT)] and alanine aminotransferase (ALT) [previously known as glutamic pyruvic transaminase (GPT)] (Fig. 2.6).

As with alkaline phosphatase, these enzymes have a wide tissue distribution. AST is found in liver, heart, skeletal muscle, kidney, brain, erythrocytes and lung. ALT has a similar distribution but activities are much lower in tissues other than the liver. The relative contributions of the particular tissues to normal serum levels are unknown, but the total activity must reflect the net effect of production and clearance. When pathological increases occur, the former will clearly be dependent not only on the nature of the cellular injury but also on the serum half-lives of AST and ALT which are known to be about 48 and 18 h, respectively. They are not cleared specifically by the kidney or by biliary excretion, but presumably enter the whole-body protein pool.

ALT is a cytosolic enzyme, whereas AST is predominantly mitochondrial ("mAST"). mAST is synthesized under control of nuclear DNA in the cytoplasm as "pre-mAST" and rapidly transferred across the mitochondrial membranes during which passage it is converted to mature mAST. mAST may be induced by ethanol and it has been suggested that the mAST/total AST ratio might be a useful diagnostic test for alcohol abuse [9] (Chapter 10).

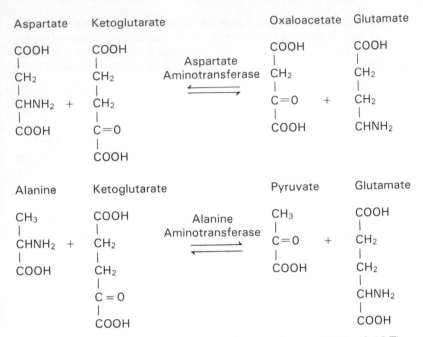

FIG. 2.6   Reactions catalysed by the aminotransferases (AST and ALT).

2.6.2.2   Basis of clinical use
The increased activities seen in patients with liver disease are presumed to originate from necrotic or damaged hepatocytes, although the necrosis is said not to be a prerequisite. It should not be assumed that the enzyme content of hepatocytes in patients with liver disease is necessarily the same as in normal hepatocytes; in patients with metastatic liver disease, hepatocyte enzyme levels may be several times higher than normal.

2.6.2.3   Use in clinical practice
The aminotransferases are sensitive tests of hepatic dysfunction [10]. This is particularly well demonstrated by the observation that during epidemics of viral hepatitis, aminotransferase levels may be markedly elevated in asymptomatic individuals. Generally speaking, the specificity of the test increases with enzyme level. Above 10 times the upper

limit of the reference range, primary hepatocyte damage is indicated so that the hepatic pathology will be some form of acute (viral or drug-induced) or chronic (such as autoimmune) hepatitis. Occasionally, acute cardiac failure or shock may cause AST levels within this range, presumably due to a combination of increased hepatic venous pressure, low cardiac output and arterial hypoxia. Exceptionally, such elevated activities may also be found in obstructive jaundice, i.e. when there is sudden acute biliary tract obstruction, or where cholangitis supervenes on biliary-tract obstruction.

Values below 10 times the upper limit of the reference range are non-specific and no aetiological inference can be drawn. Again more discrimination can be gained by considering the aminotransferase levels in relation to the ALP measured at the same time. Serum AST activity is only modestly raised in patients with alcoholic hepatitis when compared with the other hepatitides, whereas the ALT activity is often more markedly elevated. An AST/ALT ratio of > 2, in a patient who appears on clinical grounds to have a hepatitic illness, strongly suggests that alcohol is implicated (Chapter 10).

2.6.3   Gamma-glutamyl transpeptidase

2.6.3.1   Physiology and biochemistry

Gamma-glutamyl transpeptidase (GGTP) is a microsomal enzyme responsible for the transfer of glutamyl groups from gamma-glutamyl peptides to other peptides or amino acids. Although like the two previously mentioned enzymes (ALP and the transaminases), GGTP is widely distributed through the body tissues, serum levels are attributable mainly to the liver isoenzyme.

2.6.3.2   Use in clinical practice

In patients with cholestasis, the activity of GGTP tends to change in parallel with alkaline phosphatase, but it is rather more sensitive. However, GGTP levels tend to rise in all forms of liver damage and hence it is of considerably less diagnostic use than is ALP. Furthermore, an elevated level is not always due to liver damage *per se*, but may be due to induction by drugs [such as phenytoin, phenobarbitone and warfarin (Chapter 9)], alcohol (Chapter 10), pancreatic and cardiac disease, and diabetes mellitus. For this reason the test is being used less as a routine method [11] with its use being reserved for two situations.

Firstly, in the presence of an elevated serum ALP activity, a concomitant elevation of GGTP activity suggests that the ALP is of liver origin. Secondly, GGTP is the best available screening test for alcohol abuse (Chapter 10). Levels are consistently elevated in alcoholic patients with liver disease, but in only about one-quarter of those without liver disease. Although levels are higher in those with liver disease, the absolute value does not correlate with the amount of alcohol consumed or the duration of drinking.

2.7 Other serum enzymes

5'-Nucleotidase (5'-NT) catalyses the hydrolysis of nucleotides. The enzyme is located mainly on the canalicular membrane and shows increased serum activities in cholestatic conditions. Its main advantage is liver specificity, no elevation being noted in patients with bone disease. However, the difficulty of the assay mitigates against routine use (account must be taken of non-specific alkaline phosphatases which catalyse similar reactions). *Leucine aminopeptidase* (LAP) hydrolyses amino acids from the *N*-terminal of several proteins, particularly leucine compounds. High LAP activities are also seen in cholestasis, but like 5'-NT it remains normal in bone disease and does not rise in childhood or adolescence, although the activities of both 5'-NT and LAP do rise steadily throughout pregnancy.

The relative merits of ALP, GGTP, LAP, and 5'-NT in terms of sensitivity and specificity for different types of liver disease have been discussed extensively. As indicated below, such arguments have been overtaken by time. The serum activities of these enzymes are no longer used in making major therapeutic decisions, but rather to indicate the most useful next test. In most centres the combination of AST, ALP and GGTP proves satisfactory.

2.8 The serum proteins

The liver is the site of synthesis of all plasma proteins except the immunoglobulins which are synthesized in the reticuloendothelial system. Serum proteins other than albumin which are important in the diagnosis of various liver diseases are considered elsewhere and include the coagulation proteins (Chapter 4), transferrin (Chapters 3 and 11), caeruloplasmin (Chapter 11) and α-1 antitrypsin (Chapter 11).

2.8.1   Serum albumin

2.8.1.1   Biochemistry and physiology

Albumin is the major circulating protein, and is synthesized exclusively in the liver. About 12 g is synthesized each day and, of the total body pool of 300 g, about 60% is in the extravascular pool and 40% in the vascular pool. The serum half-life is 21 days and the liver is probably the major site of breakdown although many other tissues are involved. Albumin is responsible for maintaining plasma oncotic pressure, and binds numerous hormones, anions, drugs and fatty acids.

Serum albumin is unusual among human proteins in that it has no glycosidic residues, being a single polypeptide chain, 573 amino acids long. Preproalbumin, the molecule synthesized on the rough endoplasmic reticulum (RER), has an additional 24 amino acid sequence which permits the nascent protein to be transferred across the RER. Removal of the first 15 amino acids results in proalbumin which then migrates to the Golgi apparatus where cathepsin B removes the final five amino acids prior to secretion of albumin into the sinusoids.

2.8.1.2   Basis of clinical use

The serum albumin level is widely regarded as an index of hepatic "synthetic function". Whilst there is no doubt that chronic liver disease may indeed result in decreased albumin synthesis and consequent hypoalbuminaemia, several other important factors influence the serum levels and must be taken into account.

(i) The rate of hepatic albumin synthesis falls rapidly in the face of inadequate protein intake — this is a frequent occurrence in patients with alcoholic liver disease and, indeed, serum albumin is often used as an indicator of malnutrition.

(ii) Even when the rate of synthesis falls, serum levels may remain constant because of a concomitant compensatory reduction in the rate of degradation.

(iii) Hypoalbuminaemia may be present in the face of normal (or even increased) rates of synthesis when the protein "leaks" into lymph, ascites or otherwise into the extravascular compartment, or the serum albumin is diluted due to salt and water retention.

(iv) There is some evidence that alcohol may inhibit albumin secretion from hepatocytes, whilst synthesis proceeds normally.

(v) Serum albumin has a long half-life (21 days) so that only chronic changes in the synthetic rate will significantly influence serum levels.

2.8.1.3 Use in clinical practice [12]

When a patient presents with liver disease, the finding of a low serum albumin is classically taken to indicate that there is an underlying chronic component or that the acute disease is relatively long-standing. This assumption would be justified if the hepatic synthetic rate was the only factor which influences serum levels. As it is, in view of the several other factors influencing the serum level, considerable caution should be exercised before reaching any conclusions about the duration of the disease process. On the other hand, it is probably because so many different factors influence the serum albumin concentration, each of which may be affected by different disease processes, that its serum level is nearly always found to be an important prognostic feature in any chronic liver condition.

A normal albumin level in a patient with cirrhosis is an indicator of good synthetic function. It has been stated that a *normal* serum albumin makes cirrhosis unlikely (less than 15% probability) [12]. This contention is almost certainly based on hospitalized patients with decompensated liver disease. The great majority of patients with cirrhosis are not in hospital and have normal albumin levels.

2.8.2 Serum globulins

As part of the standard LFT profile it is customary to estimate the total serum globulin fraction as the difference between total protein and albumin. The individual globulins are referred to elsewhere (Chapter 6). Any fall in serum albumin tends to lead to a compensatory rise in the globulins, but extreme elevations ($> 50 \, \mathrm{g} \, \mathrm{l}^{-1}$) are usually only seen in autoimmune liver disease.

2.9 Prothrombin

Over the years, the prothrombin time has achieved the status of honorary LFT and, as such, its role is considered briefly here. A more detailed account is given in Chapter 3.

2.9.1 Physiological and biochemical basis

Quick's one-stage prothrombin time measures the rate at which prothrombin is converted to thrombin in the presence of thrombo-plastin, calcium and other coagulation factors. In turn, the thrombin leads to the conversion of fibrinogen to fibrin (Chapter 3). Prothrombin and factors VII, IX and X all require vitamin K to become active.

2.9.2 Basis of clinical use

In the presence of liver disease a prolongation of the prothrombin time indicates either poor utilization of adequate supplies of vitamin K due to parenchymal liver disease, or low serum levels of vitamin K due to obstructive jaundice. The latter situation is remedied by parenteral vitamin K (10 mg), and a rapid (within 24 h) return to normal by the prothrombin time may thus be taken as evidence of an obstructive lesion.

2.9.3 Use in clinical practice

A prolonged prothrombin time in a patient with chronic liver disease indicates advanced disease and is a poor prognostic feature (see Section 2.13). When the prothrombin time is prolonged by > 3 s there is said to be an increased risk of haemorrhage after liver biopsy and it is conventional to try to correct the prothrombin time with fresh frozen plasma before performing the procedure. In patients with acute hepatitis, or who have taken an overdose of paracetamol (Chapter 9), an increasingly prolonged prothrombin time may herald the development of fulminant hepatic failure; conversely, return towards normality is a sign of impending recovery.

2.10 Use of LFT profiles in differential diagnosis

In current practice the clinician wishing to assess liver function requests (or receives) a battery of several, rather than single, test results. The pattern of abnormalities therein provides information additional to that provided by the individual tests. Thus having described these individual tests in some detail the practical aspects of recognizing characteristic patterns of LFTs in different clinical situations is now considered. It is not uncommon for textbooks to give tables or diagrams of the values of various LFTs in different diagnostic categories. This is misleading; in any condition the tests are not static but change with time and treatment. It is more useful to consider the tests in certain distinct clinical situations:

  (i) at the time the patient first presents — when the LFTs may offer clues which help to establish a diagnosis;

  (ii) monitoring response to therapy or disease progression. Here the diagnosis has been established — one is no longer concerned with the specificity of the test, but rather its implications for the current status of the patients' liver function;

  (iii) certain of the LFTs may help towards establishing a prognosis;

  (iv) the clinician may be faced with abnormal LFTs in a patient in whom hepatic disease was not suspected — the test having been undertaken as a screening procedure.

2.11 LFTs and the differential diagnosis of jaundice

The development of jaundice is a dramatic sign and its differential diagnosis presents a challenging clinical problem. Having dealt with the congenital hyperbilirubinaemias (Section 2.5) and jaundice of haemolytic origin (Section 2.4) we now consider hepatocellular and cholestatic jaundice, the latter being subdivided into intra- and extra-hepatic causes. The distinction is not always clear cut, and in individual cases there is nearly always some degree of overlap. Nonetheless, the classification forms a practical approach on which management decisions can be made.

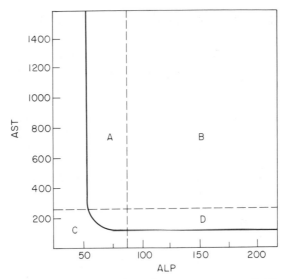

FIG. 2.7 Diagnostic value of serum enzyme activities in the differential diagnosis of jaundice. A diagrammatic representation of the relation between ALP and AST in 145 patients with either acute viral hepatitis or obstructive jaundice. The curve represents the line on which the results for most patients fall. Compartments B and C are non-diagnostic [but contain 85 (59%) of the patients]: 93% of those in A had hepatitis, and 91% of those in D had obstructive jaundice. (Adapted from Clermont and Chalmers [10].)

2.11.1 Cholestasis and cholestatic jaundice [13]

The term cholestasis implies failure of biliary secretion. Used strictly it indicates that the failure of secretion lies at the level of the hepatocyte, but it is more practical to broaden the definition to include any obstruction to bile flow occurring between the hepatocyte and the gut.

Bile is secreted across the canalicular domain of the hepatocyte plasma membrane. The canaliculus is sealed by the "tight junctions", but these can be crossed by water and inorganic ions — the paracellular pathway. The remainder of the plasma membrane, the "baso-lateral" and sinusoidal domain contains the Na^+, K^+-ATPase activity. Bile formation is the result of several transport processes occurring at the baso-lateral membrane (uptake), within the hepatocyte (intracellular transport) and across the canalicular membrane (secretory processes). Intrahepatic cholestasis may presumably be caused by lesions at any or all of these sites.

Thus in cholestasis there is a tendency for all substances secreted in the bile to accumulate in the serum, although levels of bilirubin do not always increase in the early stages of the disease process, hence the need to distinguish between cholestasis and cholestatic jaundice. The other characteristic biochemical correlates are bilirubinuria (even in the absence of jaundice), and elevation of alkaline phosphatase, GGTP and 5'-NT levels to a greater degree than the amino-transferases. Serum bile acid concentrations (Chapter 3) are also greatly increased as are cholesterol and triglyceride levels. In addition to jaundice the major clinical correlates are pruritus (which may precede the appearance of jaundice by several weeks); pale stools (due to absence of bile pigments), and dark urine (due to conjugated bilirubin in the urine).

Extrahepatic cholestasis refers to mechanical obstruction some-where between the bifurcation of the hepatic duct and the point at which the duct enters the duodenum. The bifurcation is, strictly speaking, intrahepatic but obstruction at this point leads to the same clinical picture as more distal obstruction. In contrast to intrahepatic cholestasis there is bile duct dilatation proximal to the lesion which is readily demonstrable by cholangiography or ultrasonography, although it should be remembered that in the presence of cirrhosis the liver may be so fibrotic that dilatation cannot occur. When present, the degree of jaundice is characteristically fluctuating if gallstones are the cause, rapidly progressive when attributable to malignancy, and slowly progressive when due to a post-operative bile duct stricture or primary sclerosing cholangitis.

The multiple causes of intrahepatic cholestasis have been listed in Chapter 1. *The conventional liver function tests do not permit distinction between intra- and extra-hepatic cholestasis*; nor do they allow a specific diagnosis to be arrived at, although other laboratory tests do help in the differential diagnosis. For example, a positive mitochondrial antibody test (Chapter 6) suggests a diagnosis of primary biliary cirrhosis in the presence of cholestasis. The major role of the conventional LFTs is to help to distinguish cholestatic from hepatocellular jaundice. Early studies suggested that concentrations of an abnormal low density lipoprotein termed *lipoprotein X* of greater than $300\,mg\,ml^{-1}$ were indicative of extra- rather than intra-hepatic cholestasis. This suggestion has not been confirmed by subsequent reports.

2.11.2 Hepatocellular jaundice and its distinction from cholestatic jaundice

The principal causes of "hepatocellular" jaundice are those conditions characterized by inflammation (the hepatitides): viral, chronic and drug-induced hepatitis. The absolute level of serum bilirubin is of little diagnostic significance but typically there is a marked increase in the aminotransferase activity with relatively normal levels of alkaline phosphatase and 5'-NT.

This contrasts with the situation in cholestasis and thus, by considering the relative activities of the transaminases and alkaline phosphatase, we can gain some idea as to whether the jaundice is of cholestatic or hepatocellular origin (Fig. 2.7). However, even when the results of these two tests are sufficiently extreme to make the distinction clear (D, Fig. 2.7), it must be remembered that there are several causes of intrahepatic cholestasis (Chapter 1) in which the lesion is not amenable to surgical intervention. Thus, even after a confident diagnosis of cholestatic jaundice based on the LFTs is made, further investigation to define the site of obstruction is imperative. *It cannot be too strongly emphasized that over-interpretation of the standard liver function tests in this respect can lead to serious mismanagement.*

On the other hand, when the LFTs and clinical features are compatible with a hepatitic illness [typically acute viral hepatitis (A, Fig. 2.7)], further investigation is not always required and a case can often be made for observing events. If this course is to be followed, it is important to understand the characteristic sequential changes that occur so that early referral for hospital investigation can be made should the expected course not ensue.

In acute viral hepatitis the serum aminotransferase levels always start to rise before the onset of jaundice, and often before hepatomegaly is detectable. Levels start to fall coincidentally with the onset of jaundice and symptoms, and return to normal (AST before ALT) at about the same time as the serum bilirubin, although it should be noted that the serum may remain jaundiced long after bilirubin can no longer be detected in the urine (see below). The alkaline phosphatase is seldom above $200 \, IU \, l^{-1}$ at presentation, but may rise much higher in that small group who enter a cholestatic phase long after symptoms have subsided. Normal values for LFTs are achieved within six months; persistence of abnormal LFTs beyond this period indicates the development of chronic hepatitis.

A very small percentage of patients with acute hepatitis of any aetiology, perhaps less than 1%, progress to fulminant hepatic failure which is strictly defined as the development of encephalopathy (which may range in severity from mild confusion to deep coma) within eight weeks of the first signs or symptoms of liver disease. The activity of the serum aminotransferases is characteristically very high, often $> 1000 \, IU \, l^{-1}$, but this is not of any prognostic importance, and patients with equally high values may not develop the syndrome. Later, whilst the patient is still extremely ill, levels may fall dramatically, although in this situation it is not a sign of recovery, but simply that very few liver cells remain to be further damaged. The bilirubin concentration rises early in the course of the disease although encephalopathy may occasionally precede the onset of jaundice which is seldom deep. Hypoglycaemia is common (Chapter 7) and may prove fatal if not treated rapidly. Renal failure is also a frequent complication (Chapter 3).

Bilirubin bound to albumin ("bili-albumin"), probably covalently, is now recognized as a third form of bilirubin. It may account for up to 90% of total bilirubin, in both hepatocellular and cholestatic jaundice, though impaired bilirubin excretion and an intact conjugating mechanism are prerequisites for its formation. It is thus not detectable in normal subjects or in patients with unconjugated hyperbilirubinaemias including Gilbert's syndrome. This is the form of bilirubin that persists in serum after it has ceased to be detectable in the urine [3, 4].

It is not possible to give a complete algorithm of how the LFT results will influence further investigations because this will depend on the history and clinical findings in the individual patient. *Indeed after a careful history and examination the LFTs will not always add further diagnostic information.* However, as a very general rule, if the picture is cholestatic, then the next step is ultrasound examination (to assess whether the intrahepatic bile ducts are dilated, and indicating a mechanical obstruction), and if hepatocellular, either to observe events if acute viral hepatitis is suspected, or liver biopsy where chronic liver disease is suspected.

2.11.3 Neonatal jaundice

Normal full-term babies may be jaundiced from the second to the eighth day of life, and premature babies from the second to the fourteenth. This "physiological" jaundice, in which the serum bilirubin concentration seldom exceeds $100 \, \mu mol \, l^{-1}$, is unconjugated

TABLE 2.2 Some of the commoner causes of conjugated hyper-bilirubinaemia in infancy. Several of these may also accentuate "physiological" unconjugated hyperbilirubinaemia

Biliary atresia
Cryptogenic
Infections, bacterial (e.g. *E. Coli*) or viral (e.g. Hepatitis B)
Genetic (e.g. $\alpha - 1$ antitrypsin deficiency or cystic fibrosis)
Endocrine (e.g. hypothyroidism)
Total parenteral nutrition

and attributable to a combination of factors: increased production and impaired uptake of bilirubin together with increased reabsorption from the gut. Jaundice detectable on the first day of life, or outside the ranges described above, is always pathological, as is conjugated hyperbilirubinaemia at any time.

If the unconjugated bilirubin (UCB) levels exceed $300\,\mu\mathrm{mol\,l^{-1}}$ in full-term infants, there is a significant risk of kernicterus (brain damage due to uptake of unconjugated bilirubin) and treatment by phototherapy or exchange transfusion is indicated. Thus, while measurement of serum bilirubin is not indicated as a routine in jaundiced neonates, it becomes crucial to the management of any neonate with deepening jaundice. Separation of conjugated and unconjugated fractions gives useful clues as to the cause of the jaundice (Table 2.2).

Kernicterus is due to uptake of UCB across the blood–brain barrier as the maximum binding capacity of the serum albumin for bilirubin is exceeded. In pre-term, low birthweight babies kernicterus may occur at lower bilirubin levels, both because of low albumin binding capacity and immaturity of the blood–brain barrier. Certain drugs such as salicylates and sulphonamides may actively displace bilirubin from the albumin molecule and hence increase the unbound fraction of UCB and the risk of kernicterus at even moderate bilirubin levels.

2.11.4 Conjugated hyperbilirubinaemia — the neonatal hepatitis syndrome

The characteristic clinical picture of neonatal hepatitis is of a jaundiced infant, usually aged less than one month, with pale stools and dark urine, often with hepatomegaly and failing to thrive. Thus the syndrome would seem to be more appropriately termed neonatal cholestasis. In reality the cause may be hepatocellular or cholestatic and it is the diagnosis of the extrahepatic causes, which are amenable to surgical correction (extrahepatic biliary atresia, choledochal cyst, and spontaneous perforation of the bile duct), which is the difficult and important task. The standard LFTs confirm the hyper-bilirubinaemia, and levels of the aminotransferases and alkaline phosphatase are elevated, but they do not provide any evidence about the level of obstruction or whether or not the jaundice is hepato-cellular.

2.11.4.1 Biochemical tests of bile-duct patency
The Rose–Bengal test has proved to be a most useful laboratory test in identifying the cases of extrahepatic obstruction. If less than 10% of an intravenously administered dose is excreted in the stools over a 72-h period this is strong evidence for extrahepatic obstruction (Chapter 11). More recently, technetium-labelled hepatobiliary imaging agents such as 2, 6-dimethylphenylcarbomylmethyliminodiacetic acid (HIDA) and PIPHIDA have been used. These tests, when combined with liver biopsy, give accurate results in the great majority of cases.

2.12 Monitoring response to therapy

Liver biopsy and sophisticated radiological tests may be very helpful in establishing a diagnosis but thereafter they are not suitable for frequent repetition to assess progress, both in view of cost and safety aspects, and it is here that the standard LFTs find their greatest use.

The changes occurring during the development and resolution of typical acute type A hepatitis have already been described (Section 2.11.2). In the case of type B (and non-A non-B) hepatitis there is a potential for progression to chronic liver disease in a small number of cases (Chapters 1 and 5). Such a course is manifested by the persistence of abnormal LFTs six months after the onset of symptoms, and is an indication for liver biopsy.

LFTs are also used to monitor the response of patients with autoimmune chronic active hepatitis to immunosuppressive therapy, whereas in those with chronic active hepatitis related to hepatitis-B infection, it is the various parameters of viral replication which are monitored (Chapter 5). Following diagnosis of autoimmune chronic active hepatitis (Chapter 6), high-dose prednisolone is administered $(15–50\,\text{mg day}^{-1})$ and this usually leads to a prompt fall in AST levels and bilirubin to the normal range within a few weeks or months. The dose of corticosteroid is then gradually reduced to between $7\cdot5$ and $12\cdot5\,\text{mg day}^{-1}$, provided that a normal AST level is maintained. Induction of remission is confirmed histologically. Any subsequent rise in AST to over three times the upper limit of the reference range is consistently associated with histological and clinical relapse though rising AST levels usually antedate symptoms and permit appropriate adjustment of the immunosuppressive therapy (Fig. 2.8). Unfortunately this approach to management is far from perfect because histologically active disease may be present despite normal LFTs.

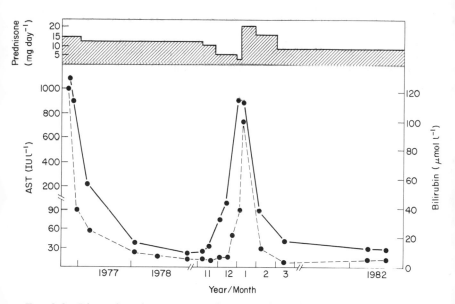

FIG. 2.8 Liver function tests used to monitor therapy in autoimmune chronic active hepatitis. Changes seen in relation to corticosteroid therapy in a 22-year-old girl. Note that during an attempt to withdraw treatment the patient relapsed and that the AST (—) rose before, and returned to normal after, the serum bilirubin (----) indicating that it is a more sensitive marker of liver damage.

Thus there is a pressing need for more sensitive tests of disease activity if reliance on frequent liver biopsies is to be avoided.

In the treatment of neoplastic liver disease selective destruction of malignant tissue is, of course, the aim. Thus, following cytotoxic chemotherapy or arterial occlusion, increases in serum AST and ALT during the week following the procedure are an indication of successful treatment (see Fig. 8.9). After surgical resection of liver tumours there is also a marked and consistent rise in AST activity (but not ALP) which lasts for a few days. When the resection is extensive the serum bilirubin concentration also rises and the albumin concentration falls. These changes are much more marked and long lasting when the patient has underlying cirrhosis.

Changes in LFTs, particularly aminotransferase levels are used to monitor new drugs for adverse hepatic reactions, although abnormalities are not always an indication for drug withdrawal (Chapter 9).* Following surgical procedures to relieve obstructive jaundice, regular measurement of serum bilirubin will aid early recognition of complications. Sudden rises in AST or GGTP in patients with alcoholic liver disease may indicate an unreported excessive alcohol consumption. Abnormal LFTs are the first sign of rejection following liver transplantation. Rejection is not diagnosed unless serum bilirubin and alkaline phosphatase are raised, and in the absence of other explanations, rejection is assumed if the AST level and prothrombin time are also rising.

2.13 LFTs as indicators of prognosis

A low serum albumin, prolonged prothrombin time and raised bilirubin are features which adversely influence survival time in patients with chronic liver disease, but the confidence limits are usually so wide that in the individual patient little significance can be attached. However, in certain situations (such as primary biliary cirrhosis and alcoholic hepatitis) more precise figures may be attainable. It has been recognized for many years that, although the prognosis of PBC is highly variable, once the serum bilirubin begins

* For example, there is an isolated rise in serum bilirubin concentration during the first month of treatment with Rifampicin but this clears spontaneously with continued administration of the drug due to its enzyme-inducing properties.

to rise the prognosis becomes worse and when the level exceeds $120 \mu mol\, l^{-1}$ survival is seldom more than two years.

Using a computer model a more accurate index has been developed, but the serum bilirubin level is still the most important factor [14] and a formula for predicting the likely outcome of patients with alcoholic cirrhosis has also been established based on the bilirubin concentration and the prothrombin time [15].

In fulminant hepatic failure, where there have been countless parameters examined with a view to identifying those patients likely to survive, serum bilirubin and the prothrombin time still appear to be the best indicators. If the serum bilirubin concentration rises above $300 \mu mol/l$ or the PT is more than 50 seconds prolonged then survival is less than 15%.

2.13.1 Child's classification (and Pugh's modification) of cirrhosis

Details of these classifications which are used to assess prognosis and operative risk, particularly after variceal haemorrhage, have been given in Chapter 1, but it should be noted again that elevated bilirubin and low albumin concentrations are features indicating a poor prognosis.

2.14 Abnormal LFTs in the absence of symptoms of liver disease

Up to 50% of patients with liver disease will already have progressed to cirrhosis before they first present with any signs and symptoms thereof, while other patients with cirrhosis may have no symptoms until malignant change develops. Furthermore, cirrhosis is not uncommonly found incidentally at autopsy. Thus it is clear that there must be a vast amount of subclinical liver disease in the population at large and it should not be surprising that, with the use of multichannel autoanalysers and health-screening programmes which provide the physician with LFTs routinely, abnormalities are being found in patients without overt signs or symptoms. Whether the therapeutic intervention offered outweighs the anxiety generated, the inconvenience and cost of consequent investigations, and implications for subsequent life assurance is not clear, but a specific diagnosis is not always achieved and, as implied above by the incidental finding of cirrhosis at autopsy, the disease detected may not cause any symptoms in the patients lifetime.

Alcohol abuse is the commonest factor implicated. The isolated finding of an abnormal AST level is usually associated with fatty liver due to obesity, often in association with diabetes or alcoholism. Less common causes include asymptomatic chronic hepatitis and haemochromatosis. The differentiation between these pathological processes can only be made on histological grounds and because they are all to some extent treatable this finding has been considered as an indication for liver biopsy [16]. Bearing in mind the previously mentioned physiological and non-hepatic pathological causes, isolated elevations of ALP are usually attributable to subclinical primary biliary cirrhosis, or metastatic tumour. Hyperbilirubinaemia due to Gilbert's syndrome will be found in about 1% of healthy individuals.

2.15 Normal LFTs in the presence of overt liver disease

Normal standard LFTs do not exclude chronic liver disease and cirrhosis. Patients with alcoholic cirrhosis who abstain from drinking, and those with well-controlled chronic active hepatitis (often at the stage of cirrhosis) may have perfectly normal tests (Chapters 1 and 6). Signs of portal hypertension (such as oesophageal varices) which are usually indications of chronic liver disease may, in the presence of normal standard LFTs, indicate extrahepatic disease such as portal vein thrombosis, although the PT is often modestly prolonged.

2.16 Interpretation of LFTs — a summary

In practice, the interpretation of LFTs will be governed by what is already known about the patient, particularly the clinical findings and

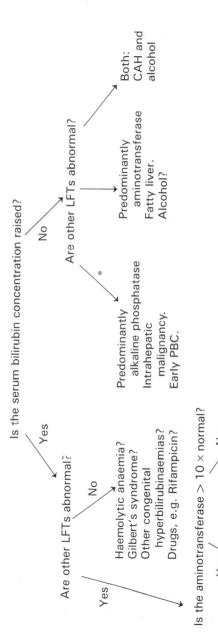
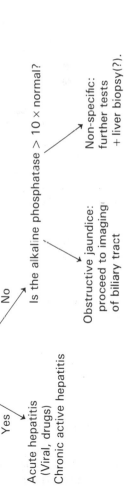

Is the serum bilirubin concentration raised?

Yes → No →

Yes branch:

Are other LFTs abnormal?

No → Haemolytic anaemia? Gilbert's syndrome? Other congenital hyperbilirubinaemias? Drugs, e.g. Rifampicin?

Yes → Is the aminotransferase > 10 × normal?

Yes → Acute hepatitis (Viral, drugs) Chronic active hepatitis

No → Is the alkaline phosphatase > 10 × normal?

Obstructive jaundice: proceed to imaging of biliary tract

Non-specific: further tests + liver biopsy(?).

No branch:

Are other LFTs abnormal?

→ Predominantly aminotransferase Fatty liver. Alcohol?

→ Both: CAH and alcohol

* → Predominantly alkaline phosphatase Intrahepatic malignancy. Early PBC.

FIG. 2.9 Interpretation of LFTs in a patient suspected of having liver disease.

* Check liver specificity—GGTP raised?

history. However, taking a hypothetical patient with suspected liver disease Fig. 2.9 offers a simple and logical approach to the analysis of the LFTs.

References

1. Sherlock S. Diseases of the Liver and Biliary System. Oxford: Blackwell Scientific Publications, 1987.
2. Schmid R. Gastroenterology 1978; 74: 1307.
3. Weiss JS, et al. New Engl J Med 1983; 309: 147.
4. Lester R. New Engl J Med 1983; 309: 183.
5. Bailey A, et al. Does Gilbert's syndrome really exist? Lancet 1977; i: 931.
6. Fevery J, Blanckaert N. J Hepatol 1986; 2: 113.
7. Berk P. In: Butterworths International Medical Reviews: Gastroenterology 4, Liver (Williams R, Maddrey WC, Eds). London: Butterworths, 1984: 1.
8. Kaplan MM. Hepatology 1986; 6: 526.
9. Lumeng L. Hepatology 1986; 6: 742.
10. Clermont RJ and Chalmers TC. Medicine 1967; 46: 197.
11. Penn R and Worthington DJ. Brit Med J 1983; 286: 531.
12. Whicher J and Spence C. Ann Clin Biochem 1987; 24: 572.
13. Scharschmidt BF, et al. New Engl J Med 1983; 308: 1515.
14. Neuberger J, et al. Transplantation 1986; 4: 713.
15. Maddrey WC, et al. Gastroenterology 1978; 75: 193.
16. Hultcrantz R, et al. Scand J Gastroenterol 1986; 21: 109.

Suggested further reading

Clermont RJ and Chalmers TC. The transaminase tests in liver disease. Medicine 1967; 46: 197–207.
Kaplan MM. Serum alkaline phosphatase — another piece is added to the puzzle. Hepatology 1986; 6: 526–528.
Lester R. Not two, but three bilirubins. New Engl J Med 1983; 309: 183–185.
Mowat AP. Liver disease in childhood. London: Butterworths, 1987.
Scharschmidt BF, Goldberg HI and Schmid R. Approach to the patient with cholestatic jaundice. New Engl J Med 1983; 308: 1515–1519.

Schmid R. Bilirubin metabolism: state of the art. Gastroenterology 1978; 74 1307–1312.

Sherlock S. Diseases of the Liver and Biliary System. Oxford: Blackwell Scientific, 1987.

3

Other biochemical tests

3.1 Introduction

There are several biochemical tests, other than those described in Chapter 1, which are either useful under special "non-routine" circumstances, or which have been proposed but not yet widely accepted, and which have not yet achieved the status of a standard liver-function test (LFT). Also considered in this chapter are the investigations appropriate for patients with ascites and renal failure.

3.2 Serum bile acids

The serum bile acids (SBAs) have for decades been the poor relation of the bile pigments in terms of their use as a diagnostic test. This, despite the fact that the acids have a distinct physiological role, whereas the pigments are "useless products of a minor metabolic pathway" [1]. The reason is, or has been, purely technical. Until recently it was extremely difficult to measure bile acids in serum accurately, but over the last decade assays have improved and sensitive methods are now available.

3.2.1 Biochemistry and physiology

Although complicated, it is important to understand the outline of the biosynthesis of bile salts and their enterohepatic circulation in order to appreciate their potential use and limitations as a diagnostic test. The bile acids are steroid molecules synthesized in the liver from the cholesterol. Cholic and chenodeoxycholic acids (CA and CDCA) are the *primary* acids. The rate-limiting step is the hydroxylation of cholesterol by the hepatic microsomal 7α-hydroxylase which is under negative feedback control being inhibited by reabsorbed bile salts (Fig 3.1). Before secretion in the bile they are conjugated with either taurine or glycine, thereby increasing solubility. After passage through the small intestine, where fat absorption is facilitated, most bile acids are actively reabsorbed from the ileum. Those reaching the large bowel are partially deconjugated and converted by the action of bacterial 7α-dehydroxylase to *secondary* bile acids: deoxycholic and lithocholic acids (DOCA and LCA), the former being of much greater quantitative importance. Deoxycholic acid and, to a lesser extent, lithocholic acid are reabsorbed to be reconjugated in the liver either with glycine or taurine. Lithocholic acid

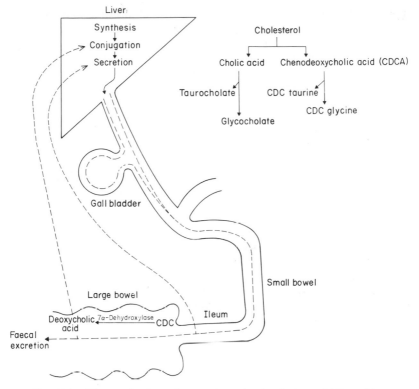

FIG. 3.1 The synthesis and enterohepatic circulation of bile acids.

undergoes sulphation as well as conjugation, a process which limits subsequent reabsorption. Therefore, there is an enterohepatic circulation, which serves to conserve effectively the bile acids — the small amount lost in the faeces (500 mg day^{-1}) being made up by synthesis in the liver. A third metabolite, ursodeoxycholate (a stereoisomer of CDCA), is found in trace amounts and has been classified as a *tertiary* bile acid.

After food, bile enters the duodenum from the gall bladder and bile acids achieve a concentration of 10–40 mmol l^{-1}, a level at which micellar aggregates form. The major physiological function of the bile salts is to permit dispersion of long-chain fatty acids into micellar solution along with other dietary lipids including the fat-soluble vitamins A, D, E and K. Bile acids are largely confined to the enterohepatic circulation, less than 1% being present in peripheral blood. In normal subjects, the level of SBAs is

51

determined by the difference between the amount absorbed from the gut, and that taken up by the liver and because the latter is probably fairly constant, it is the amount absorbed from the gut which determines the serum levels. Under pathological conditions, however, the hepatic clearance becomes important. This is itself dependent on liver blood flow and the degree of portosystemic shunting.

3.2.2 Serum bile acids as a test of liver function

Kits are now commercially available which permit SBAs to be measured with confidence. These include enzymatic methods, radio-immunoassays (RIAs) or assays based on bioluminescence and measure total non-sulphated bile acids or cholyglycine or sulphated lithocholic acid conjugates. The reference range for total SBAs, measured by an enzymatic technique is $0·5-8\,\mu\text{mol}^{-1}$ in the fasting state rising to $6-11\,\mu\text{mol}^{-1}$ 2 h after food. Serum bile acids are elevated in most patients with chronic liver disease because there is a failure of hepatic uptake due to a combination of hepatocellular dysfunction and portosystemic shunting.

Dissatisfaction with the standard LFTs has led to intensive investigation of the possible role of measurements of bile acid concentrations either absolutely or as ratios of one another, as tests of liver function. However, new tests such as these undergo far more intensive assessment before being introduced into clinical practice than did the standard LFTs.

From the mass of available data it appears safe to conclude that elevated levels of SBAs are remarkably specific for the presence of liver disease, the exception being bacterial overgrowth of the small intestine. It is worth noting that, in the presence of ideal dysfunction, the enterohepatic circulation will be disrupted and normal levels will be found even in the presence of liver disease. The test is less sensitive in detecting liver disease, and in particular aspartate amino-transferase (AST) is a more sensitive test of mild liver disease and, contrary to early reports, there seems to be no advantage of post-prandial sampling (2 h after a meal) over fasting samples. Calculation of the area under the time–concentration curve after a meal increases the sensitivity, but the time and effort involved limits wide application. The test permits good distinction between mild and severe chronic active liver disease — an important clinical distinction because the latter benefits from treatment — but the degree of overlap is such that liver biopsy can still not be avoided.* Overall there seems to be little justification for the routine use of these tests in the diagnosis of hepatobiliary disease [2–4].

3.3 Clearance tests: towards a quantitative evaluation of liver function [5,6]

These tests quantitate the ability of the liver to clear certain exogenous compounds from the body and are sometimes referred to as 'dynamic' liver function tests.

3.3.1 Pharmacological basis and practical requirements

Ideally, the test compound should be eliminated mainly or exclusively by the liver, non-toxic, and readily measurable.

$$\text{Clearance} = \text{hepatic removal/arterial plasma concentration}$$

$$\text{Hepatic removal} = \text{plasma flow} \times (\text{arterial} - \text{venous concentration})$$

Thus,

$$\text{Clearance} = \text{plasma flow} \times \frac{(\text{arterial} - \text{hepatic venous})}{\text{arterial}} \text{ concentration}$$

Thus clearance is a function of plasma flow and, the second term in this equation, the *hepatic extraction ratio*, E. When the extraction ratio approaches 1, the clearance equates with liver blood flow. In normal subjects, the value of E for indocyanine green (Section 3.3.2), for example, is about $0 \cdot 9$ so that the clearance is a measure of blood flow. However, in the diseased liver, E may fall as low as $0 \cdot 2$ and the clearance becomes dependent on the functional capacity of the liver.

This test is thus claimed to measure the functional hepatic mass (FHM). This concept, borrowed from renal medicine, assumes firstly that each liver cell has the same functions as the whole liver and that

---

* In patients with cirrhosis who have a normal AST value, fasting bile acid levels are consistently raised, leading to the suggestion that SBAs could be a "second level" test in patients suspected of cirrhosis in whom conventional tests are normal or borderline.

the FHM therefore equals the function of one cell multiplied by the total number of cells. Secondly, it is assumed that all cell functions vary in parallel so that two cells with 50% function are equivalent to one with 100% function.

Compounds such as aminopyrine, antipyrine and caffeine, have extraction ratios of less than 25% in normal subjects, and provided saturating doses of these agents are given, their clearance is largely independent of blood flow and may be considered to be a measure of functional hepatic mass.

3.3.2   The indocyanine green test

Indocyanine green is taken up solely by the liver and excreted unchanged, without conjugation. It is non-toxic, apart from very occasional urticarial reactions. The dose administered to assess functional hepatic mass is $5 \, \text{mg kg}^{-1}$ and samples are taken between 3 and 15 min. The percentage disappearance rate (PDR) is then simply calculated as:

$$PDR = 0 \cdot 693 / t_{1/2} \times 100$$

where $t_{1/2}$ is the half-life of indocyanine green. In normal adults the initial disappearance rate is between 17 and 22%, and figures below this are considered abnormal.

3.3.3   The bromsulphthalein test

Bromsulphthalein (BSP) is a cholephilic dye which after intravenous injection is bound to albumin, taken up by hepatocytes and conjugated with glutathione before biliary excretion. After a standard dose of $5 \, \text{mg kg}^{-1}$, serum samples are taken at 5-min intervals for 45 min and the concentration calculated by measuring the extinction at 580 nm after addition of 20% potassium hydroxide. The results are best plotted on semi-logarithmic paper and, from the resultant curve, the slope of the two exponential curves can be calculated. The slope of the second exponential component, K_2, is a measure of hepatic excretory function. Values below 3% min^{-1} are considered abnormal. A simplified form of the test is based on a single reading at 45 min and expressed as a percentage assuming an initial plasma concentration of $10 \, \text{mg ml}^{-1}$. Unfortunately, BSP occasionally causes an anaphylactoid reaction and phlebitis and its use has now been largely superseded by indocyanine green.

3. OTHER BIOCHEMICAL TESTS

3.3.4 The galactose elimination capacity [7]

As for BSP the index compound, galactose, is administered intravenously and samples for blood galactose concentration are taken over
1 h. The results may be analysed in terms of a clearance (as above), but
the relation between V_{max} and the half-life is very complex. It is more
satisfactory to calculate the galactose elimination capacity (GEC) over
the initial 15 min during zero order clearance.

$$GEC = (m - u)/(t_{C=0} + 7)$$

Where m is the dose injected, u is the amount excreted in the urine
over the next 4 h and $t_{C=0}$ is drug concentration at time 0 by
extrapolation of the curve to the abscissa. The value of 7 min
compensates for the fact that the blood concentration is lower than
the concentration in the volume of distribution (Fig 3.2).

3.3.5 The aminopyrine breath test [8]

This test, like antipyrine and caffeine clearance, is a quantitative test

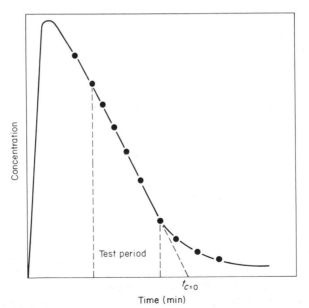

FIG. 3.2 The determination of the galactose elimination capacity.

of microsomal function based on hepatic clearance of radiolabelled aminopyrine measured by the concentration of CO_2 in the breath. An oral dose of $1 \cdot 5$–2 U μCi $[^{14}C]$-aminopyrine dissolved in water is administered orally. Breath samples are then collected in a trapping solution of ethanol and hyamine at fixed times, either multiple samples at half-hour intervals or a single sample at 2 h, and counted in a liquid scintillation spectrometer. The result is expressed as a percentage of the total dose administered.

Patients with severe parenchymal liver disease have a decreased fractional excretion and this is predominantly attributable to a decreased functioning hepatic mass, as the extraction ratio of aminopyrine is low and clearance is little changed by the altered hepatic blood flow.

3.3.6   What is the role of the dynamic liver function tests?

Why is it that, despite all the well recognized inadequacies of the standard LFTs and the good evidence that clearance tests really do give an overall estimate of liver function, none of these tests is used widely in clinical practice? Problems with individual tests are mentioned above, but, in general, clinicians do not perceive that enough information is gained in relation to the effort required to undertake the test. *A priori*, the major role of such tests would seem to be in determining prognosis, but in most clinical situations the physician is only required to give a very rough opinion of a patient's prognosis, and he recognizes that functioning hepatic mass can be only one factor in an overall equation. There are, however, two clinical situations in which these tests may became more widely used.

First, with the increasing availability of liver transplantation it is becoming important to determine as accurately as possible a patient's prognosis in comparison with the risks associated with transplantation. Clearance tests may have a role to play here, although in one recent small study of the prognostic importance of the $[^{14}C]$-amino-pyrine breath test, the test performed poorly and was inferior to serum albumin [7]. Second, there are several conditions in which the natural history is so prolonged (primary biliary cirrhosis, for example) that to determine the effect of new treatments on survival would take decades. If tests for liver function improvement which could predict subsequent prolongation of survival were available, this would indeed be a valuable advance.

The problem with all biochemical tests of liver function is that there is no accepted "gold standard'. New tests tend to be compared with older ones and circular arguments ensue. Histological examination is, at present, the nearest to a "gold standard" available, but why this should be is far from clear particularly in view of the subjective nature of the test and extreme vulnerability to sampling error. However, it is clear that in this situation no test can be better than liver biopsy. It seems likely that the use of biochemical tests will remain an art rather than a science for the foreseeable future.

3.4 Investigation of hepatic encephalopathy: ammonia and amino acids

The measurement of blood and cerebrospinal-fluid (CSF) ammonia has a long and distinguished history in liver disease. This is because it has been considered to play a central role in the pathogenesis of liver coma. Whether or not this is so remains an area of great controversy at the present time and here we must confine discussion to the extent to which measurement may be useful from a diagnostic point of view.

A major role of the liver is to defend the brain against noxious nitrogenous compounds originating in the gut. In patients with cirrhosis, portal hypertension may lead to portosystemic shunting where portal blood enters the systemic circulation directly, bypassing the liver and reaching the brain. Hence the term portal–systemic encephalopathy (PSE). Many different compounds are probably responsible, together with increased sensitivity of the brain, but ammonia has been the most widely studied. In most patients with encephalopathy, CSF and serum levels of ammonia are raised, and fall during recovery, although the first signs of encephalopathy often occur before blood ammonia starts to rise [9].

Measurement of blood ammonia is less used nowadays. Firstly, accurate measurements are time consuming and require very careful handling of specimens. Secondly, it is usually clinically obvious that encephalopathy is due to liver disease and the course of the illness can be monitored easily without ammonia estimation.

Patients with PSE characteristically exhibit increased concentration of the aromatic amino acids (such as phenylalanine and tyrosine) and reduced concentration of the branched-chain amino acids (leucine, isoleucine and phenylalanine). The major interest in these findings lies in relation to the pathogenesis of hepatic encephalopathy and these tests are not used routinely for diagnostic purposes.

The ammonium tolerance test involves administering an oral dose of 3 g ammonium chloride and measuring arterial ammonium at 45 min. A rise of more than $150 \mu g \, dl^{-1}$ is abnormal and indicative of porto-systemic shunting [11].

3.5 Serum tests of hepatic fibrosis

Measurement of fibrosis which is a characteristic feature of chronic liver disease and responsible for several of the complications thereof, has received little attention until recently. The only accurate method of assessment was histological examination of liver tissue and other tests, such as serum or tissue prolyl hydroxylase, are technically difficult. Recently, there has been considerable interest in immunological methods for the assay of aminoterminal procollagen type-III peptide (PIIIP) [10].

3.5.1 Aminoterminal procollagen type-III peptide

Procollagen peptides are globular proteins which are cleaved from the ends of the procollagen molecule by procollagen endopeptidases to leave the helical part of the molecule to grow further. Commercial kits are now available to measure serum PIIIP and it is apparent that the test shows promise both diagnostically and in monitoring progression of disease and response to treatment. Strictly speaking the level appears to reflect fibrogenesis (i.e. the rate of ongoing fibrosis) rather than the absolute amount of fibrosis. In particular, levels are high in alcoholic hepatitis (but not fatty liver) and decline after withdrawal of alcohol. Likewise, levels are higher in patients with chronic active hepatitis than chronic persistent hepatitis. The test is, at present, still of interest mainly as a research tool.

3.6 Biochemical changes during the formation of ascites and the development of renal failure

The pathogenesis of ascites and renal failure which are both frequent complications of advanced liver disease is complex and controversial.

Nonetheless, laboratory investigation plays a crucial role in establishing a diagnosis in both conditions (which often co-exist), and in monitoring response to treatment.

3.6.1 Ascites

Ascites, the excessive accumulation of extracellular fluid in the peritoneal cavity (over 30 l in some cases), is usually a late complication of cirrhosis. The precise mechanism is still argued over, but the primary event is probably sodium retention (due in part to secondary hyperaldosteronism), compounded by hypoalbuminaemia and localized to the peritoneal cavity by portal hypertension. Thus the urine may become virtually sodium free and, so long as sodium intake exceeds output, fluid will continue to accumulate [12]. Ascites usually develops in patients with advanced, decompensated disease, but the tendency to retain salt is present before ascites actually develops, and a sudden increase in dietary salt intake may lead to ascites which spontaneously clears when the salt intake is restricted. There are, however, several liver and non-liver diseases other than cirrhosis which can lead to the formation of ascites (Table 3.1) and the establishment of a precise diagnosis is important for its correct management.

If the routine LFTs are abnormal, then it is likely that one of the liver diseases listed in Table 3.1 is responsible and it is often already known that the patient developing ascites has cirrhosis. However, patients with liver disease can develop ascites for reasons other than

TABLE 3.1 Causes of ascites: conditions in bold type are frequently associated[a]

Primary hepatic disease	Non-hepatic disease
Cirrhosis	**Abdominal malignancy**
Budd–Chiari syndrome	**Cardiac failure**
Portal vein thrombosis	**Constrictive pericarditis**
Acute, and sub-acute liver failure	Peritonitis (especially tuberculous)
	Malnutrition
	Pancreatic disease

[a] A large ovarian cyst, filling the abdomen, can often be confused with ascites but liver function tests are normal.

cirrhosis. For example, patients with alcoholic cirrhosis may develop tuberculous ascites, pancreatic ascites and also "malignant" ascites if hepatocellular carcinoma supervenes. Cardiac causes can usually be diagnosed confidently on clinical grounds, but the other causes may be difficult to distinguish and laboratory investigation can be useful here. Using a needle, it is easy to perform a so-called "diagnostic tap", to obtain ascitic fluid for analysis. The investigations and their interpretation are shown in Table 3.2. It should be recognized that sodium retention is not a diagnostic feature of cirrhotic ascites; equally intense sodium retention is seen in "malignant" ascites.

The figures for ascitic protein given in Table 3.2 can offer no more than a rule of thumb [13]. There are so many exceptions to the rules that many would consider the test useless. However, as the changes become more extreme, so their diagnostic specificity increases. Thus a protein concentration below $10\,\mathrm{g\,l^{-1}}$ is not infrequent in uncomplicated cirrhosis, but virtually rules out malignant disease. Conversely, protein concentration above $35\,\mathrm{g\,l^{-1}}$ are the rule in malignant ascites.

3.6.2 Monitoring treatment of ascites

Ascites due to cirrhosis is usually managed by a combination of dietary-salt restriction and diuretic therapy, though paracentesis with albumin infusion is now being used more widely. It is often forgotten that the aim is simply to relieve the patient's discomfort and improve his appearance; ascites does little harm of itself. It is thus important not to make the patient feel worse with over-enthusiastic treatment.

The aim should be to achieve a net fluid loss of $500\,\mathrm{ml\,day^{-1}}$, until the ascites clears. Serum urea, creatinine and electrolyte concentrations should be checked at least once a week at the start of treatment. A rising serum urea or creatinine and falling serum sodium concentration ($<130\,\mathrm{mmol\,l^{-1}}$) indicate impending renal failure and should lead to reduction of diuretic treatment. Serum creatinine concentration is the more useful test as impaired urea synthesis in patients with cirrhosis make the serum urea a less sensitive indicator of renal function. Serum potassium needs careful monitoring if frusemide is used because of the risk of hyokalaemia, which may precipitate encephalopathy. Hyperkalaemia may occur with spironolactone if renal failure supervenes.

TABLE 3.2 Differential diagnosis of ascites based on inspection and tests of the ascitic fluid. So-called pancreatic ascites exhibits high concentrations of amylase (greater than the serum value) but this is a rare cause of asites, virtually confined to patients with alcoholic cirrhosis. The presence of malignant cells, detected by cytological methods, is diagnostic of malignant ascites, but such cells are only detected in a small percentage of patients with malignant ascites

	Direct inspection	Protein $(g\,l^{-1})$	Cells	Bacteria
Uncomplicated cirrhosis	Clear	< 25	$< -500\,mm^{-3}$ (mononuclear cells)	None
Intra-abdominal malignancy	Clear	> 25	Malignant cells [and (?) red blood cells]	None
Tuberculous peritonitis	Turbid	> 25	White cells (mainly lymphocytes)	Acid-fast bacilli
Abdominal lymphoma	Chylous			None

3.6.3 Spontaneous bacterial peritonitis (SBP) [14,15]

Spontaneous bacterial infection of ascites usually leads to fever, rigors and colicky abdominal pain, together with hepatic decompensation, but in up to one-third of cases the peritonitis may be silent and the only indication is progressive deterioration of hepatic dysfunction.

Definitive diagnosis rests on isolation of an organism from the ascitic fluid but culture takes time and Gram's stain may be misleading. Typically, the ascitic fluid is turbid with a white cell count of $>1000 \, \text{mm}^3$, a low protein concentration ($<25 \, \text{g} \, \text{l}^{-1}$) and an arterial/ascitic pH gradient of >0.1, but these changes are not diagnostic and it may be life-saving to start treatment before the results of culture are available. Blood should be placed directly into blood culture bottles at the bed side. Antibiotics should be administered whenever there is a compatible clinical picture and the ascitic fluid contains more than 250 polymorphonuclear leucocytes per mm or more than 500 white cells per mm^3 in the absence of clinical features. The organisms most frequently implicated are *E. Coli* and pneumococcus which may also be grown from blood cultures in about 50% of cases.

The major differential diagnosis is "nonspontaneous" bacterial peritonitis due to bowel perforation. Here the white cell count is very high (often $>10\,000 \, \text{mm}^3$), and multiple organisms including anaerobes are often found. It occurs much less frequently than SBP.

3.7 Renal failure

The onset of renal failure is indicated by rising levels of serum creatinine and urea and usually, but not always, a urinary output falling to less than 300 ml day^{-1}. A particularly lethal complication, as already mentioned, is hyperkalaemia. Such developments are likely to precipitate encephalopathy in patients with liver disease.

The major clinical problem in such patients is an idiopathic form of renal failure which is widely known as the "hepatorenal syndrome" (see below) and usually associated with advanced disease, ascites and encephalopathy. This should not be confused with several other situations in which renal disease and liver disease coexist: polycystic disease, infections such as leptospirosis, circulatory failure, and the immune complex glomerulonephritis associated with hepatitis B virus infection. Renal failure may also develop when cirrhotic patients are fluid depleted, and following surgery to relieve obstructive jaundice. The latter syndrome is caused by acute tubular necrosis, but the mechanism is unknown.

3.7.1 The hepatorenal syndrome (HRS) [16]

This condition is also known as functional renal failure (FRF). The characteristic feature is that if the kidney is examined histologically it is found to be normal, i.e. there is disturbance of function but not of structure, and the usual appearances of acute tubular necrosis are not seen. Furthermore, the failure is progressive and not reserved by fluid repletion suggesting that this is not simply a "pre-renal" type failure. The precise pathogenesis is unknown, but the immediate factor is an intense renal vasoconstriction leading to decreased renal blood flow and a reduced glomerular filtration rate. It occurs classically in patients with advanced chronic liver disease but may also occur in severe acute liver disease.

The condition can be diagnosed by simple laboratory tests, reduced urine flow, and rising levels of serum urea and creatinine are common to all forms of renal failure. However, the characteristic feature of FRF, which distinguishes it from acute tubular necrosis, is the dramatic degree of sodium retention. The urinary sodium concentration is usually less than $10 \, mmol \, l^{-1}$ and often less than $5 \, mmol \, l^{-1}$. The urine/plasma osmolality is > 1. This contrasts with patients with acute tubular necrosis in whom the urinary sodium concentration is greater than $12 \, mmol \, l^{-1}$ and often greater than $20 \, mmol \, l^{-1}$ and the urine/plasma osmolality is about 1

TABLE 3.3   Differential diagnosis of renal failure in cirrhosis

	Pre-renal failure	Functional renal failure	Acute tubular necrosis
Urinary sodium ($mmol \, l^{-1}$)	< 10	< 10	> 20
Urine : plasma osmolality	> 1·15	1·10–1·15	< 1·10
Response to volume expansion	Yes	No	No

References

1. Lester R. New Engl J Med 1983; 309: 183
2. Ferraris R, et al. Dig Dis Sci 1983; 28: 129.
3. Hoffmann A. Hepatology 1982; 2: 515.
4. Fromm H and Albert MB. Gastroenterology 1987; 92: 829.
5. Branch RA. Hepatology 1982; 2: 97.
6. Preisig R. In: Recent Advances in Hepatology. 1987: 1.
7. Tygstrup N. Acta Med Scand 1964; 175: 281.
8. Henry DA, et al. Dig Dis Sci 1985; 30: 813.
9. Ansley JD, et al. Gastroenterology 1978; 75: 570.
10. Hahn EG. J Hepatol 1984; 1: 67.
11. Conn HO. Gastroenterology 1961; 41: 97.
12. Wilkinson SP et al. Clin Sci 1978; 56: 169.
13. Sampliner RE and Iber FL. Am J Med Sci 1974; 267: 275.
14. Wyke RJ. Gut 1987; 38: 623.
15. Hoefs JC, et al. Hepatology 1982; 2: 399.

Suggested further reading

Arroyo V, Gines P, and Rodes J. Treatment of ascites in patients with cirrhosis of the liver. J Hepatol 1986; 2: 504–512.

Branch RA. Drugs as indicators of hepatic function. Hepatology 1982; 2: 97–105.

Hahn EG. Blood analysis for liver fibrosis. J Hepatol 1984; 1: 67–73.

Hoffmann A. The aminopyrine demethylation breath test and the serum bile acid levels: nominated but not yet elected to join the common liver tests. Hepatology 1982; 2: 515–517.

Papper S. Hepatorenal syndrome. In: The Kidney in Liver Disease, Epstein M, Ed. New York: Elsevier Biomedical, 1983.

Paumgartner G. Serum Bile Acids. Physiological Determinants and Results in liver disease. J. Hepatol 1986; 2: 291–298.

Wilkinson SP and Williams R. Ascites, electrolytes and renal disorders. In: Liver and Biliary Disease (Wright, Millward-Sadler, Alberti and Karran, Eds.) London: Baillière Tindall, 1985.

4

Haematology

4.1 Introduction

The liver plays a central role in the maintenance of normal haematopoiesis and haemostasis. Whilst in adults the bone marrow is primarily responsible for the production of the red cells, platelets and granulocytes, subsequent red cell breakdown and bilirubin synthesis occurs principally in the liver (Chapter 2). In early foetal life, however, the liver is also the site of haematopoiesis and may become so again in adult life when bone marrow function is compromised. All the coagulation factors and their inhibitors are synthesized by the liver, as are the serum-binding proteins for iron, and vitamin B_{12} which, together with folic acid, are all stored in the liver.

To this extent it is predictable that liver disease will lead to haematological problems including disturbances of haemostasis and abnormal numbers and function of the formed elements of blood. In addition, however, in liver disease there are inhibitors of chemotaxis and neutrophil abnormalities [1]. These may lead to an increased susceptibility to bacterial infection, which is not directly related to disturbances of the known haematological functions of the liver. Patients with primary haematological disease, and others receiving blood transfusions, are at risk of contracting viral hepatitis therefrom, and jaundice, usually the province of the hepatologist, is a symptom of ineffective erythropoiesis and haemolytic anaemia.

4.2 Abnormalities of haemostasis [2]

Patients with liver disease are prone to easy bruising, bleeding after venepuncture, and nose bleeds. In liver failure, spontaneous haemorrhage into vital structures may ensue, and variceal haemorrhage may be more difficult to arrest when coagulation factors are deficient. Despite the fact that bleeding problems are only occasionally severe, assessment of the clotting factors may be useful as indicators of liver function, and as a guide to the likelihood of bleeding after invasive procedures such as percutaneous liver biopsy.

4.2.1 Physiology and biochemistry [3]

The mechanism by which blood clots only at the appropriate place and time, and the consequent lysis of the clot are extremely complex. Here, only those aspects relevant to the tests used in liver disease are considered in any detail.

Damage to blood vessels sets in motion a complex sequence of enzymatic reactions which convert inactive circulating molecules into active forms which finally result in the formation of a clot consisting of a fibrin framework and platelets. This "cascade" (Fig 4.1) is initiated either by contact of the blood with subendothelial collagen (the so-called intrinsic pathway) or by the release of thromboplastin (the extrinsic pathway) at the site of vascular damage. Both these pathways lead ultimately (via the common pathway) to the conversion of prothrombin to thrombin which, in turn, converts fibrinogen to fibrin. Polymerized fibrin forms the framework of the clot. All the factors involved are synthesized by the liver (Table 4.1). The coagulation cascade is controlled by inhibitory factors (see below), and by clearance of activated coagulation factors by the liver.

Clots are broken down by the fibrinolytic system. Plasminogen, which is synthesized by the liver, is activated by several factors including streptokinase

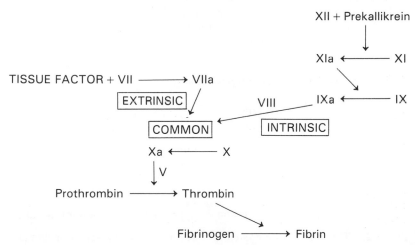

FIG. 4.1. A simplified diagrammatic representation of the coagulation cascade ('a' indicates activated factors).

TABLE 4.1. Blood-coagulation factors and their inhibitors

Number	Name
I	Fibrinogen
II	Prothrombin
III	Tissue factor (thromboplastin)
IV	Ca^{2+}
V	Proaccelerin
VI	—
VII	Proconvertin
VIII	Antihaemophilic factor
IX	Christmas factor
X	Stuart–Prower factor
XI	Plasma thromboplastin antecedent
XII	Hagemen factor
XIII	Fibrin-stabilizing factor

The protease inhibitors
  Antithrombin III
  Protein C
  Heparin cofactor 2

to form plasmin which digests fibrin leading to the formation of fibrin degradation products (FDPs) (Fig 4.2). Plasmin, together with α_2-macroglobulin, protein C and antithrombin III (AT III) are natural inhibitors of coagulation. AT III is the most powerful inhibitor and is present in decreased concentration in patients with liver disease.

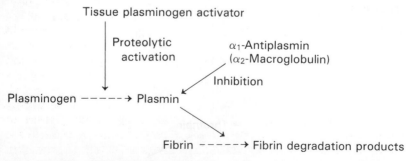

FIG. 4.2. The fibrinolytic system. Tissue plasminogen activator initiates fibrinolysis by binding to fibrin as the clot forms. Plasmin dissolves the fibrin *in situ*, but is rapidly neutralized by α_1-antiplasmin.

As part of the investigation of liver disease it is possible to measure the concentrations of the individual clotting factors. More often, tests, such as the prothrombin time (Section 4.2.3), which measure the cumulative effect of a number of factors at the same time are used.

4.2.2 The importance of vitamin K

Vitamin K is present in most vegetables (K_1) and is also formed in the gut by bacteria (K_2). Being a fat-soluble vitamin, effective absorption from the gut requires bile salts and thus when there is cholestasis, vitamin K levels fall rapidly particularly because body stores are small. Four of the coagulation factors, prothrombin (II), VII, IX and X, are synthesized in the liver in precursor form and have no coagulant activity until modified by vitamin K. Hypovitaminosis K thus results in a prolongation of the prothrombin time (PT) (Section 4.2.3).

If an abnormal PT "corrects" (i.e returns towards normal) after parenteral administration of vitamin K, it may be assumed that the defect was due to vitamin K deficiency, and implies that some degree of cholestasis was present. On the other hand, if the abnormal PT persists after vitamin K administration, then deficiency of one or more of the coagulation factors due to poor hepatic synthetic function may be assumed. In practice, 10 mg of vitamin K is given parenterally and the PT measured again between 12 and 24 h later. If the PT returns to normal, or improves by at least 50%, then the initial prolongation can be attributed to hypovitaminosis K and some degree of cholestasis assumed. Of course there are several conditions such as primary biliary cirrhosis where both cholestasis and hepatocellular damage are present and in these instances no conclusions can be drawn if a prolonged PT fails to correct.

Great progress in understanding the mechanism of vitamin-K action has been made recently [3]. Vitamin K carboxylates the 10 terminal glutamic acid residues of the vitamin K dependent coagulation precursors prior to glycosylation and secretion. This results in the formation of a unique amino acid, γ-carboxyglutamic acid, which confers coagulant (and metal binding) activity on the precursor proteins. It is of interest that, even in the presence of adequate vitamin K, decarboxylated forms of prothrombin can be detected in serum of patients with liver disease by immunological methods, although they have no coagulant activity [4]. This is particularly so in patients with hepatocellular carcinoma where des-γ-carboxyprothrombin is a useful serum marker, (Chapter 8).

4.2.3 The prothrombin time and other coagulation tests

The quick one-stage test measures the rate at which prothrombin is converted to thrombin in the presence of activated clotting factors, calcium and thromboplastin. The PT will screen for deficiencies in the levels of the plasma factors involved in the extrinsic and common pathways, i.e factors VII, V, and X, prothrombin (II) and fibrinogen (I). The normal prothrombin time is between 12 and 16 s, although each time the test is performed a normal control is included and the result expressed either as a ratio [The International Normalized Ratio (INR)] of the patients' time to the normal control, or in "seconds prolonged", again in relation to the normal control. Prolongation of more than 3 s (or INR > 1·2) is usually considered abnormal.

Assuming (as the test does) that the plasma fibrinogen level is normal ($> 50 \, \text{mg ml}^{-1}$), then a prolonged PT suggests either: (i) a deficiency (< 30% normal) of one of the four factors involved — this may be congenital (for example, "Christmas disease", where factor IX is deficient); or (ii) as is the case in liver diseases, acquired — as discussed above in patients with liver disease the prothrombin time will be prolonged either when there is deficiency of any of the four factors involved in the test, or of vitamin K. Severe protein malnutrition may also lead to a deficiency of the clotting factors; or (iii) the presence of specific inhibitors of one of these factors (such as the anticoagulant drug, warfarin); or (iv) high concentrations of fibrin degradation products.

4.2.3.1 The partial thromboplastin time
The partial thromboplastin (PTT) test is the standard test for the integrity of the *intrinsic* common pathways (Fig 4.1; Section 4.2.1). For the investigation of the patient with liver disease this test adds a little further information to the PT, although it is frequently used together with the PT.

4.2.3.2 The thrombin time
The thrombin time is sensitive to decreased levels of fibrinogen, the presence of fibrin(ogen) degradation products and abnormal fibrinogen molecules "dysfibrinogenaemia".

4.2.4 Implications of a prolonged prothombin time in liver disease

In acute hepatitis, a prolongation of the PT of more than 5 s defines a group of patients at an increased risk of progressing to acute (fulminant) liver failure (FHF). However, even within this group few will progress to FHF and only when the PT is prolonged by more than 50 s does this, by itself, indicate the need for referral to a specialist unit. In patients with FHF, the prothrombin time is the best single, widely available, prognostic indicator, but even here it is difficult to quantitate the risk associated with a particular value. Certainly when the PT is prolonged by more than 100 s survival is most unusual. Similarly, in chronic liver disease a prolonged PT in the absence of hypovitaminosis K, indicates poor parenchymal function and a poor prognosis (see Child's classification, Chapter 1).

4.2.5 Disseminated intravascular coagulation

Disseminated intravascular coagulation (DIC) is an haemorrhagic syndrome in which inappropriate initiation of the coagulation cascade leads to widespread intravascular coagulation, "consumption" of circulating coagulation factors and platelets, and a consequent fibrinolytic process. It is characterized by (i) low platelet count; (ii) damaged red cells (schistocytes); (iii) low fibrinogen concentration; (iv) prolongation of the thrombin time, PT, and PTT; and (v) high titres of fibrin(ogen) degradation products.

The diagnosis in patients with liver disease is difficult because many of these abnormalities are present for reasons other than DIC, and many patients appear to have a chronic low grade DIC of no clinical significance. The only clinical situation that appears to be regularly associated with DIC occurs when ascites is treated by reinfusion into the systemic circulation [5].

When the thrombin time is prolonged but the concentration of FDPs and fibrinogen is normal, an *acquired dysfibrinogenaemia* should be suspected. This is present in up to 75% of patients with liver disease and caused by an increased amount of sialic acid in the carbohydrate side chains of the fibrinogen molecule [6].

4.2.6 The risk of haemorrhage after needle liver biopsy [7]

It is normal clinical practice to measure the prothrombin time (and group, and cross-match two units of blood before percutaneous needle biopsy of the liver is undertaken. If the former is prolonged by more than 3 seconds (INR > 1·2), or if the platelet count is less then $80 \times 10^9 l^{-1}$ (or $60 \times 10^9 l^{-1}$ if hypersplenism is present (Section 4.3.2)) the procedure is deferred. Treatment with vitamin K (Section 4.2.2), platelet transfusion or fresh frozen plasma, as appropriate, may reverse the abnormalities for a sufficient time that the procedure can be carried out safely. Where it is essential to obtain a histological diagnosis and PT or platelet count remain outside the acceptable range even after replacement therapy, a transjugular liver biopsy may be performed (entering the liver by the hepatic vein). This technique requires a very experienced operator and is still not without risk.

As with all invasive procedures entailing risk to the patient, the decision to proceed or not should depend on the ratio of risk to benefit for the patient rather than absolute laboratory figures. Many physicians remain to be convinced that the PT is really an important way of predicting likely haemorrhage following biopsy, and likewise it is probably the functional capability of the platelets rather than their absolute number that is crucial. Significant haemorrhage (i.e. that requiring treatment — there is probably always some minor degree of bleeding) is very rare. The mortality rate, which is invariably due to haemorrhage, is approximately 10 cases per 100 000 [8], and usually seen with inexperienced operators and/or in patients with advanced disease particularly malignancy and obstructive jaundice.

4.2.7 Abnormalities of specific clotting factors

Several families with the Dubin–Johnson syndrome have been described who have isolated factor VII deficiency which is not corrected by the administration of vitamin K [9]. Low concentrations of factors V and VII appear to be correlated with a poor hepatocellular function and hence a poor prognosis. Neither are widely used as prognostic tests in clinical practice.

Concentrations of factor VII are increased in liver disease and this may be helpful in distinguishing between coagulopathy due to fulminant hepatic failure (when factor VIII levels are very high) and DIC (Section 4.2.5) where factor VII levels are low, due to consumption.

4.2.8 The Budd–Chiari syndrome

Thrombosis of the hepatic venous system is a rare but serious event leading to ascites and liver failure. In some cases it is associated with an overt myeloproliferative disease such as polycythaemia rubra vera or paroxysmal nocturnal haemoglobinuria (PNH) but in about one-third of cases no cause is found [10]. PNH may be diagnosed by a positive Ham's test or sucrose haemolysis test, both of which rely on the extreme susceptibility of patients' red cells to complement mediated haemolysis *in vitro*. Recently a number of cases have been reported in which the "lupus" anticoagulant was detectable [11]. Paradoxically, this is associated with an increased tendency to clotting and is suspected when the activated partial thromboplastin time and kaolin clotting time are prolonged. Based on measurement of serum erythropoietin levels and bone marrow erythroid progenitors it now appears that polycythaemia may not always be primary but, rather, a transient response to increased hepatic erythropoietin production [12].

4.3 The full blood count

As with the liver function tests (LFTs), the clinician usually receives a battery of tests when a full blood count is requested. This usually comprises at least, the red-cell, white-cell, and platelet counts, the haemoglobin concentration together with the various red cell parameters including mean corpuscular volume (MCV), blood film and a differential white-cell count. The haematinics, iron, folic acid and vitamin B_{12} are all stored in the liver. The liver stores about 1 mg of vitamin B_{12} in total (which is sufficient to last for several years) and about 5 mg of folic acid. Daily requirements of folic acid are greater than for vitamin B_{12} and stores only last a few months when dietary intake is compromised. Iron is stored in the form of haemosiderin or ferritin. The latter is detectable in the serum where its concentration is proportional to the total body iron stores (Chapter 11).

4.3.1 Anaemia and abnormalities of the red blood cells (Table 4.2)

Anaemia is common in patients with liver disease and its cause is

TABLE 4.2. Diagnosis of anaemia in chronic liver disease: many of the causes co-exist so that mixed pictures are common

Type of anaemia	Red-cell morphology	Marrow Examination	Se Iron	TIBC	Trans. sat.[a]	Ferritin	Vit. B₁₂	Folate	Causes
Iron deficiency	Hypochromic Microcytic	Normocellular. No iron in macrophages. Few sideroblasts	↓	↑	↓	↓	N	N	Gastrointestinal blood loss: peptic ulceration; variceal bleeding
Megaloblastic	Normochromic Macrocytic Hypersegmented neutrophils	Increased cellularity. Megaloblastic changes in erythrocyte precursors	N	N	N	N	N	↓	Folic acid deficiency due to alcoholism
Haemolytic	Macrocytes Target cells Acanthocytes Reticulocytosis	Erythroid hyperplasia	N	N	N	N	N	N	Zieve's syndrome. Wilson's disease. Autoimmune CLD
Of chronic disease	Normochromic Normocytic	Decreased/increased iron in RE cells	↓	↓	↓	N	N	N	Chronic liver disease
Aplastic	Pancytopaenia	Hypocellular, fatty	N	N	N	N	N	N	Acute viral hepatitis. Azathioprine. Cytotoxic agents
Sideroblastic	Hypochromic	Increased iron "ring sideroblasts". Megaloblastic	↑	↑	↑	N	N	↓	Alcohol

[a] Trans. sat., transferrin saturation (%).   N, normal.

multifactorial. However, to some degree the "anaemia", as measured by the haemoglobin concentration or packed cell volume (PCV), may be apparent rather than real because blood volume is often increased in patients with cirrhosis. Thus, whilst the circulating red cell mass may be normal, the haemoglobin concentration and PCV will be low. In addition there is the normochromic normocytic anaemia which can be seen in any chronic disease.

4.3.1.1 Iron-deficiency anaemia

Microcytic anaemia is seen in patients who are losing blood and it may be compounded by poor dietary intake of iron. The site of blood loss is usually the gut: either from oesophageal varices or peptic ulceration both of which frequently complicate chronic liver disease (Chapter 1). There may be fresh blood in the stool, melaena, or faecal occult blood testing may be required for its detection.

4.3.1.2 Macrocytosis and megaloblastic anaemia [13]

An elevated MCV and macrocytes on the blood film are very common in patients with liver disease and/or suffering from alcoholism (Chapter 10). Two distinct causes need to be distinguished. First, there is the idiopathic "macrocytosis of alcoholism and liver disease" which is the most common cause, and secondly there is megaloblastic anaemia due to dietary folate deficiency which occurs invariably in alcoholics, particularly spirit drinkers. Beer contains about 15 μg of folic acid compared to less than 1 μg (per 100 g alcohol) for spirits.

"Idiopathic" macrocytosis (MCV in the range 100–110 fl) occurs in up to 60% of patients with chronic liver disease and/or those suffering from alcoholism. It may be a consequence of abnormal serum lipid profiles which alter the structure of the red cell membrane, or a prolonged cell-cycle time during which the cell continues to grow. The macrocytes are described as being thin ("leptocytes") and although the MCV is high, the mean corpuscular haemoglobin concentration (MCHC) is normal. There is no associated anaemia and serum and red cell folate and vitamin B_{12} levels are normal. The MCV has been proposed as a screening test for occult alcoholism (Chapter 10). Macrocytosis is also a side effect of the drug azathioprine which is used in the treatment of chronic active hepatitis and following liver transplantation.

Excessive alcohol consumption
(especially spirits, and poor diet)
↓
Negative folate balance
↓
Low serum folate and red-cell folate
↓(one month)
Megaloblastic anaemia----→Macrocytosis and megaloblastic marrow changes
↓ (low vitamin B_6 levels)
Sideroblastic anaemia----→Ring sideroblasts in bone marrow
↓ Abstention from alcohol and normal diet
Erythroid hyperplasia and reticulocytosis
↓
Normal blood film and marrow

FIG. 4.3. Stages in the development of and recovery from the anaemia associated with chronic excessive alcohol consumption.

In alcoholic patients, however, dietary deficiency of folate is frequent and, soon after levels of serum and red cell folate fall, both macrocytosis and a megaloblastic anaemia develop (Fig. 4.3). Associated findings are hypersegmented neutrophils, a mild unconjugated hyperbilirubinaemia, and megaloblastic myeloid and erythroid precursors in the bone marrow. Among alcoholics with megaloblastic anaemia, about half will have low serum folate levels and more than 80% will have reduced red-cell folate levels. Vitamin B_{12} levels are usually normal but pernicious anaemia may co-exist and it is probably worthwhile estimating serum vitamin B_{12} levels in all patients with megaloblastic changes.

4.3.1.3 Sideroblastic anaemia
After prolonged folate deficiency, sideroblastic changes develop with a hypochromic anaemia despite normal or elevated serum iron and transferrin saturation. Sideroblastic anaemia is characteristically seen in patients with alcoholism particularly when vitamin B_6 deficiency co-exists [14] (Fig. 4.3).

4.3.1.4 Haemolytic anaemia
This is an occasional complication of patients with primary biliary cirrhosis or autoimmune chronic active hepatitis (when Coomb's test

is positive) and alcoholic patients with Zieve's syndrome [15,16]. The latter comprises acute haemolysis, unconjugated jaundice, increased serum lipids and cholesterol in a patient with alcoholic liver disease. Such cases with true acute haemolysis are rare. Many patients with chronic liver disease have a low-grade chronic haemolysis which is of little clinical importance. Reticulocytosis often occurs after stopping heavy alcohol consumption and thus does not necessarily imply haemolysis.

It is apparent from the above that alcoholism is a major factor in haemolytic anaemia. The most appropriate investigations for alcoholic patients with anaemia are, MCV, reticulocyte count, serum ferritin, peripheral blood film and red cell folate. If there are more than 3% "thick macrocytes", the MCV is greater than 110 fl, there is neutrophil hypersegmentation or the red cell folate concentration is low, then folic acid should be given if vitamin B_{12} deficiency has been excluded. A normal red cell folate level does not exclude folate deficiency and folate therapy should still be given if other factors suggest deficiency.

4.3.1.5 Aplastic anaemia

Aplastic anaemia is a very rare, but often fatal, complication of acute viral hepatitis. Patients receiving azathioprine as an immunosuppressive agent or cytotoxic agents for hepatic malignancy may also become aplastic if the dose is not monitored carefully and altered appropriately.

4.3.2 Hypersplenism

Patients with chronic liver disease often have enlarged spleens and this is invariably associated with some degree of pancytopaenia and the platelets and granulocyte counts in particular are often low. The mechanism is not fully understood, but is probably a combination of sequestration of the blood cells, increased plasma volume [17] and some degree of haemolysis. It is not infrequent to see platelet counts well below $50 \times 10^9 \, 1^{-1}$, a level at which, under other circumstances, is associated with a high risk of spontaneous haemorrhage. However, in patients with hypersplenism this type of pancytopaenia usually causes the physician far more anxiety than the patient, and although splenectomy (or portocaval shunt) may be effective in "improving" the blood count, it is very seldom needed. The operative risks usually outweigh any benefit to the patient.

The exception to this rule is in the case of isolated splenic vein thrombosis. Here splenectomy will cure both the hypersplenism and the associated portal hypertension. Treatment of patients with autoimmune liver disease with azathioprine may cause a similar pancytopaenic picture to that seen in hypersplenism. In these patients it is extremely difficult to determine to what extent a low platelet count is due to hypersplenism or marrow suppression. This is of considerable importance because the former is relatively benign and the latter potentially fatal.

4.3.3 Thrombocytopaenia

Platelets play an important role in primary haemostasis by adhering to any site of damaged vascular endothelium. Low platelet counts, which compound the haemorrhagic tendency seen in liver disease, are usually caused by alcohol toxicity. This leads to decreased platelet survival and inhibition of megakaryocyte production by the bone marrow. Folate deficiency has also been implicated. Hypersplenism (Section 4.3.2) and DIC (Section 4.2.5) are other causes already referred to. In patients with autoimmune chronic active hepatitis, antiplatelet antibodies may be present. Platelet function, as judged by the bleeding-time and platelet-aggregation tests, is also abnormal in patients with alcoholic liver disease.

4.3.4 White blood cells and their function [1]

The high risk of bacterial infection in patients with chronic liver disease is related to disturbances in the function rather than in the number of granulocytes, except when levels are very low following treatment with azathioprine or cytotoxic agents. There are defects in opsonization (the process whereby micro-organisms are coated with immunoglobulin and/or complement so as to be recognized by neutrophils as foreign), and serum factors which inhibit chemo-attractant activity. In acute liver disease, particularly fulminant hepatic failure, decreased complement levels may account for the high frequency of bacterial infection.

4.4 Other haematological abnormalities

Erythrocytosis, with haemoglobin concentrations of $> 20\,g\,dl^{-1}$ occurs in about 5% of cases of hepatocellular carcinoma in the Far East. Lupus erythymatosus (LE) cells may be seen in the peripheral blood of patients with autoimmune chronic active hepatitis (Chapter 6). "Target cells", probably an exaggerated form of the macrocyte of chronic liver disease (Section 4.3.1.2), in patients with any type of liver disease and atypical lymphocytes are not uncommon in patients with acute viral hepatitis.

4.5 Screening blood donated for transfusion

In most countries all donated blood will be screened for HBsAg (Chapter 5) and samples found positive discarded. This has led to a marked decrease in the incidence of post-transfusional hepatitis B, but the problem of non-A non-B (NANB) hepatitis remains (Chapter 5). It is likely that serological tests for the NANB viruses will be forthcoming in the near future, but in the meantime a more empirical approach has been adopted. It appears that if blood containing anti-HBc, or which has a high activity of alanine aminotransferase, is discarded then the incidence of NANB hepatitis virus infections can be decreased [18].

This approach is impractical in countries in which hepatitis B carriage is common where up to 25% of the population may be seropositive for anti-HBc. Here simultaneous administration of immune globulin at the time of transfusion may be effective in stopping the development of NANB hepatitis.

References

1. Rajkovic IA and Williams R. Clin Sci 1985; 68: 247.
2. Jackson CM and Nemerson Y. Ann Rev Biochem 1980; 49: 765.
3. Wallin R and Martin LF. J Clin Invest 1985; 76: 1879.

4. Blanchard RA, *et al*. New Engl J Med 1981; 305: 242.
5. Harman DC, *et al*. Ann Int Med 1979; 90: 774.
6. Soria C, *et al*. Thromb Res 1980; 19: 29.
7. Sherlock S, *et al*. J Hepatol 1984; 1: 75.
8. Piccinino F, *et al*. J Hepatol 1986; 2: 165.
9. Seligshohn U, *et al*. Quart J Med 1974; 39: 569.
10. Poewell-Jackson PR, *et al*. Quart J Med 1982; 51: 79.
11. Van Steenbergen W, *et al*. J Hepatol 1986; 3: 87.
12. Levy VG *et al*. Hepatology 1985; 5: 858.
13. Lindenbaum J. Sem Liver Dis 1987; 3: 169.
14. Eichner ER and Hillman RS. Am J Med 1971; 50: 218.
15. Pengelly CDR and Jennings RC. Postgrad Med J 1971; 47: 683.
16. Zeive, L. Ann Int Med 1958; 48: 471.
17. Lieberman FL and Reynolds TB. J Clin Invest 1967; 46: 1297.
18. Holland PV. In: Viral Hepatitis 1981 International Symposium (Szmuness W, Alter HJ, Maynard JE (Eds)). Philadelphia: Franklin Institute Press, 1981: 563.

Suggested further reading

Jackson CM and Nemerson Y. Blood coagulation. Ann Rev Biochem 1980; 49: 765.

Kelly DA and Tuddenham ECG. Haemostatic problems in liver disease. Gut 1986; 27: 339–349.

Lindenbaum J. Hematologic complications of alcohol abuse. Sem Liver Dis 1987; 3: 169–181.

Rajkovic IA and Williams R. Mechanisms of abnormalities in host defences against bacterial infection in liver disease. Clin Sci 1985; 68: 247–255.

5

Virology

5.1 Introduction

Viral infections are the commonest cause of acute hepatitis in man. The range of responsible viruses is very broad but the most important epidemiologically are the A, B and Delta viruses and (increasingly) the so-called non-A, non-B (NANB) group. The A and B viruses were originally distinguished as separate entities by the differences in their modes of transmission, the lengths of their incubation periods and their respective clinical sequelae. Hepatitis A (infectious hepatitis) (i) is transmitted via the faecal–oral route, (ii) has a relatively short incubation period (generally 3–6 weeks) and (iii) patients usually successfully eliminate the virus during the acute phase and chronic infections seem not to occur. In contrast, hepatitis B (serum hepatitis) (i) is transmitted mainly through blood-to-blood contact (although other routes, e.g. via saliva, or semen between sexual partners, are also important), (ii) tends to have a longer incubation period (up to three months, occasionally longer), and (iii) can lead to a chronic carrier state (with or without underlying liver damage).

The true incidence of acute hepatitis throughout the world is not known, because infection can present simply as flu-like illnesses without jaundice and remain undiagnosed. However, the World Health Organization estimates that there are about 200 million carriers of the hepatitis B virus worldwide. The highest prevalence is among the peoples of Asia, Africa, South America and countries bordering the Mediterranean Sea, but pockets of endemic infection also exist in Europe and North America (mainly among the homosexual and drug-addict communities) and in other countries.

During the past 30 years, much progress has been made in our understanding of the hepatitis A and B viruses and a battery of specific serological tests for these viral infections is now available. With the advent of these, and of tests for other agents known to cause hepatitis, it became apparent that there is another group of hepatitis viruses that had until fairly recently remained unknown. These viruses have still not yet been identified but their existence is now beyond doubt and, for obvious reasons, they have been termed the NANB viruses. Developments in hepatitis virus serology are continuing so rapidly that it is difficult to keep pace but the "state of the art" presented here is as up-to-date as is possible within the technical constraints of publication.

5.2 Hepatitis A virus (HAV)

The hepatitis A virus (HAV) is a 27-nm RNA enterovirus of the picornavirus sub-group. The usual mode of transmission via the faecal–oral route occurs mainly through personal contact (especially among children but also between sexual partners), the drinking of contaminated water, or the consumption of shellfish (especially filter feeders, such as clams and other bivalves, that concentrate the virus) from sewage-contaminated waters. HAV is ubiquitous in its distribution and appears to be antigenically identical throughout the world. The mechanisms of liver damage in HAV infection are not fully understood. The virus may be cytopathic, but hepatocellular injury might also be due to host immune reactions against virus-infected cells and/or to virus-induced autoimmune reactions.

After infection, the virus replicates in the liver during the incubation period. A low-grade viraemia develops, reaching a peak just before the onset of symptoms and disappearing rapidly as the clinical illness commences (Fig. 5.1). At this time also, virus particles are shed in the stools. *De novo* infections elicit a *primary* (IgM) antibody response that begins at the onset of symptoms and continues with rising titres during the acute phase (Fig. 5.1). Titres of IgM anti-HAV fall rapidly during recovery and patients usually become seronegative for this antibody within a few weeks. However, not infrequently, the IgM anti-HAV persists at a lower level, which might reflect prolonged acute (and, therefore, still potentially infectious) disease. Shortly after the onset of symptoms, the *secondary* (IgG) antibody response begins to develop. Titres of IgG anti-HAV continue to rise for several

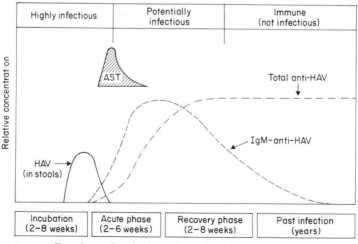

FIG. 5.1.   Serological events in HAV infection.

months after recovery. Thereafter, they may decline to a lower level, but subjects usually remain seropositive for life and this antibody seems to provide protection against re-infection. Thus the diagnostic serology for HAV infection is the finding of IgM anti-HAV in the patient's serum, the IgG antibody being a reflection of past infection.

5.3 Hepatitis B virus (HBV)

The hepatitis B virus (HBV) is one of a group of Hepadna viruses that infect man and other animals. In northern countries, horizontal transmission of HBV via the parenteral route used to occur mainly during blood transfusion or injection of blood products, but the development of screening programmes to identify HBV-positive blood donors has led to a marked reduction in the number of infections acquired in this way and careful monitoring of HBV-positive mothers and therapeutic intervention in the newborn is beginning to reduce vertical (maternal/foetal) transmission. In these countries, infection is now largely confined to certain high-risk groups, e.g. drug addicts, homosexuals, bisexuals, individuals receiving multiple blood transfusions and/or whose immune systems are compromised, and institutionalized subjects (the mentally handicapped and prison inmates). Other cases of HBV infection in these areas seem to arise mainly through close contact (e.g. via skin abrasions) or between heterosexual partners (the virus is present in vaginal secretions, semen, saliva and most other body fluids). Elsewhere, vertical transmission is probably the most important factor in maintaining the high level of infection in the population, for neonates who acquire the virus almost always become chronic carriers. However, the possibility that vectors such as mosquitoes and other biting insects may play a role in transmission cannot be excluded.

HBV seems not to be inherently cytolytic [1] and hepatocellular injury appears to be related to the host's immune reactions against virus-infected liver cells and possibly also to a concomitant virus-induced autoimmune response (Chapter 6). It is generally thought that there is only one type of HBV that infects humans. Worldwide this has a common specificity, "a", on the coat protein envelope (Fig. 5.2) but several sub-types (ad, ar, aw, ay) are known. Infection with one sub-type confers protection against infection with other sub-types. Other hepadna viruses, although closely related to HBV, are found only in animals (notably the North American woodchuck and ground squirrel and the Pekin duck). Recently, however, what appears to be a new hepatitis B virus infecting children in Senegal has been described [2]. The

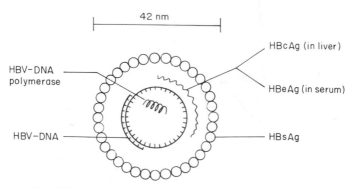

FIG 5.2. Schematic representation of the complete hepatitis B virion (Dane particle).

putative new virus is very similar to HBV in that it produces an acute hepatitis with HBs-antigenaemia, and chronic carriage occurs, but it differs from HBV in its core antigen and there is no appearance of the usual HBV markers, HBeAg, anti-HBe, anti-HBc or anti-HBs in the serum (see below).

5.3.1 HBV serum markers

The complete HBV virion (Dane particle) is a 42-nm particle with a circular DNA core surrounded by a protein coat (Fig. 5.2). The virus carries its own specific DNA polymerase enzyme which it uses to replicate itself. Electron-microscopic examination of sera collected during an acute infection reveals numerous particles of different sizes. In addition to the 42-nm particle, there are 22-nm spheres and rod-like structures which vastly outnumber the full virus particles. These represent excess coat protein which the virus produces in copious amounts. This material was the first serum marker of HBV infection to be identified and was originally called "*Australia antigen*" (because it was discovered in the blood of an Australian aborigine) but is now known as "*hepatitis B surface antigen*" (*HBsAg*).

A second marker is a protein, known as the "*core*" *antigen* (*HBcAg*), that is intimately associated with the virus DNA (Fig. 5.2). This is not usually detected in the blood because it is normally complexed to anti-HBc antibody (see below) but a very closely related protein, the "*e*" *antigen*, which is probably derived from HBcAg by proteolytic cleavage [3], can be detected in serum and is almost always associated with the presence of the complete virion. The finding of

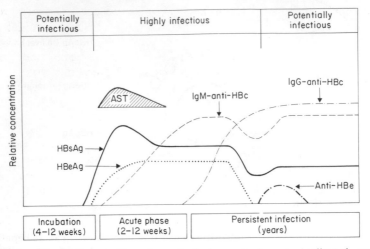

FIG 5.3. Classical sequence of serological events in uncomplicated acute hepatitis B.

HBeAg in the serum therefore indicates that the patient is highly infectious (Fig. 5.3).

In addition to screening for HBsAg and HBeAg, progress of the infection can be monitored by the detection of serum antibodies (anti-HBs and anti-HBe) reacting with both of these antigens as well as with HBcAg (i.e. anti-HBc).

A number of other serological markers of HBV infection have been identified. These include the virus DNA genome (HBV-DNA) and its specific DNA polymerase, which are more sensitive indicators of continuing active viral replication than is HBeAg. Techniques for detecting these two markers in serum are becoming commercially available and either or both may eventually replace several of the other markers currently in use.

Two other markers are currently receiving considerable attention. These are antibodies against a specific part (pre-S) of the surface coat protein and against the receptor for polymerized human serum albumin (pHSA). The pre-S component is in two parts, pre-S_1 and pre-S_2. The latter contains the pHSA receptor (pHSAr), which is believed to be important for the attachment of the HBV virion to the hepatocyte in order to facilitate its entry to the cell. IgM-anti-pre-S can be detected before HBsAg in the serum [4]. Commercial kits have now been developed for these markers and when fully evaluated they may be added to the battery of tests for HBV infection, especially for monitoring individuals receiving the new generation of recombinant HBV vaccines containing pre-S components (see Section 5.8).

5.3.2 Serological sequelae in typical acute HBV infection

The sequence of events that occur with respect to the appearance and disappearance of the various serum markers in uncomplicated acute HBV infection is depicted in Fig. 5.3. In contrast to HAV infection, the viraemia which develops during the prodromal phase usually reaches a peak shortly after the onset of symptoms and can be demonstrated serologically by the finding of HBsAg and HBeAg, as well as HBV-DNA and HBV-DNA-polymerase. Disappearance of the full virus particles from the blood begins during the acute phase, usually before the peak in serum aminotransferase levels, and patients typically become HBeAg-negative as symptoms subside. At or about the onset of symptoms, the virus elicits a primary (IgM) antibody response to the "core" protein (HBcAg) and IgM-class anti-HBc antibodies begin to appear in the blood and rise in titre during resolution of the illness. During this period, however, large quantities of the "coat" protein (HBsAg) continue to be produced by the infected liver and HBsAg may persist in the blood for several weeks after recovery but with declining titres.

As viraemia wanes (with the disappearance of HBsAg), antibodies (anti-HBe) to the "e" antigen begin to appear in the serum and may continue to rise for several months. This switch from HBe anti-genaemia to anti-HBe production is known as *seroconversion* and it heralds a period during which the patient becomes progressively less infectious. Complete confidence that the patient is no longer infectious, however, comes only with the disappearance of HBsAg and appearance of anti-HBs. At this point, a secondary (IgG) antibody response to HBcAg begins, coinciding with the gradual reduction in the titre of IgM-anti-HBc. IgG-anti-HBc titres rise to a plateau and then slowly decrease, but the antibody usually remains with the patient for life.

5.3.3 Atypical serological sequelae

There are numerous variations in the sequence of events described above. These seem to depend partly on the host's immune response to the infection and partly on the dose of virus received, but other factors, such as the route of transmission (e.g. blood transfusion or sexual contact), may also be important.

From the clinical standpoint, the two variations that are most worthy of note are: (i) the development of the carrier state (see below), and (ii) the patient who is strongly suspected of having an HBV infection but is found to be seronegative for HBsAg and HBeAg. The latter situation can arise when the viraemia is short-lived and peaks before the onset of symptoms (Fig. 5.4). Often, the clinical impression can be confirmed by demonstrating anti-HBe and/or anti-HBs in the serum and, because the majority of patients with HBV infections will have one or more of these four serum markers (HBsAg, HBeAg, anti-HBe, anti-HBs), these are the tests that most routine laboratories will perform.

Occasionally, the antibody responses will be slow to develop and a patient may be found to be seronegative for all four markers for a time. This period is known as the "*core window*" and the only evidence of HBV infection will be the presence of IgM-anti-HBc in the serum (Fig. 5.4). The "core window" may, however, be only artefac-

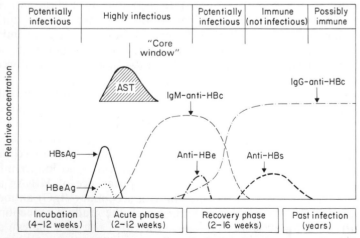

FIG 5.4. Atypical sequence of serological events in uncomplicated acute hepatitis B.

tual because the recent development of highly sensitive tests for anti-HBs detection, based on the use of monoclonal antibodies, has revealed that many of the patients exhibiting this phenomenon do have low titres of anti-HBs that are undetectable by the less sensitive methods.

5.3.4 The carrier state

A proportion of subjects infected with HBV become chronic carriers—defined as persistence of HBsAg in the blood *for more than six months*. In Europe and North America, only about 1% of patients who develop acute HBV hepatitis fail to clear the virus, but in areas where HBV is endemic it is thought that the proportion who become carriers may be as high as 10%. The term "carrier" derives from early studies identifying these individuals among blood donors, but is somewhat misleading. "Chronic infection" is perhaps a more apt description because a significant proportion of such individuals will have chronic liver disease of varying severity, including many who are apparently healthy with normal liver function tests (see Section 5.7.2).

Perinatally acquired infection probably accounts for the majority

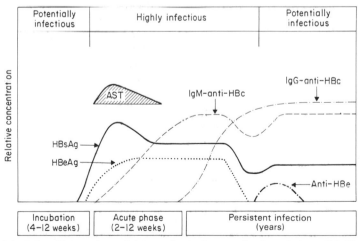

FIG 5.5. Illustration of the serological events in chronic hepatitis B following an acute infection. Note: seroconversion from HBeAg to anti-HBe may occur after a few months or years (as shown) but HBeAg may persist for life.

of HBV carriers worldwide, but the chronic infection can commence with an acute hepatitis. This is often mild and may even be sub-clinical, but the symptomatic phase, when it occurs, may be somewhat protracted (2–3 months or longer). At this stage, the serology is typical of early acute HBV infection, i.e. positive for HBsAg, HBeAg and also often for IgM-anti-HBc (Fig. 5.5). However, these markers then persist and the patient remains infectious. Persistence of HBsAg and HBeAg without development of anti-HBe or anti-HBs may last for life but often patients will seroconvert from HBeAg to anti-HBe at some stage (six months to several years after infection), remaining seropositive only for HBsAg and anti-HBc and presenting a lower infectious risk. Seroconversion is sometimes accompanied by what, clinically and biochemically, appears to be a second episode of acute hepatitis and may be related to Delta virus superinfection (see below).

5.4 Hepatitis Delta virus (HDV)

The hepatitis Delta virus (HDV) was first detected by Rizetto in 1977. It is a defective pathogen with an RNA genome and a specific protein (the Delta antigen, HDAg) enclosed within an envelope of *HBV* surface protein (HBsAg). All of the evidence to date indicates that it is wholly dependent on HBV and is acquired by the same routes, either as a *co-infection* with the initial HBV inoculum or as a *super-infection* in a person who is already carrying HBV. Thus it occurs only in individuals who are infected with HBV. Persons who are immune to HBV (e.g. vaccinees with circulating anti-HBs antibodies) are pro-tected from Delta virus infection.

The distribution of Delta virus around the world varies greatly, even within areas where HBV is endemic. The highest prevalence recorded (83%) was among chronic HBV carriers in Roumania. The incidence in patients with acute or chronic HBV infections ranges from 10% to 50% in Mediterranean countries and the Middle East but is surprisingly low in other areas where HBV is endemic, such as India, mainland China, most parts of Russia, the Pacific Islands (with a few notable exceptions) and the southern half of South America. In northern parts of South America (notably the Amazon basin, northern Columbia and western Venezuela), however, the Delta virus is endemic and gives rise to a particularly severe form of acute hepatitis variously known as *Black Fever*, *Labrea hepatitis* or *Santa Marta hepatitis* [5]. The Delta virus is virtually non-existent in Japan and among the Eskimos and North American Indians, while elsewhere in North America and in northern Europe, Delta infections are so far largely confined to persons with frequent blood contacts (drug addicts, haemophiliacs). In these areas, it is surprisingly uncommon among homosexuals, but some spread to the general HBV-infected population is becoming evident. Vertical (maternal/foetal) transmission seems to be relatively unimportant in maintaining endemicity of Delta virus, but there is considerable evidence of *horizontal* intra-familial transmission by close body contact.

Delta virus infection may be acute or chronic. The sequence of events depends to some extent upon whether the virus is acquired as a co-infection or as a super-infection. *Co-infection* can lead to a biphasic acute hepatitis with a periodicity of up to six weeks in which the first episode is due to HBV and the second to the Delta virus. Unless specific tests for Delta virus are performed (see below) this second episode may be misinterpreted as a relapse of the HBV-induced illness. In uncomplicated cases, the second episode is commonly accompanied by clearance of HBV and, therefore, also of the Delta virus.

Super-infected HBV carriers may experience a self-limiting hepatitis followed by clearance of Delta virus and sometimes also of HBV. More often, the initial acute Delta hepatitis in a super-infected individual is followed by chronic hepatitis. It seems that the presence of the Delta virus is associated with a more rapid progression to cirrhosis (and consequently a poorer prognosis) and it has been suggested that the Delta virus may be responsible for a proportion of those apparently healthy HBV carriers who, on investigation, are found to have on-going liver damage.

5.4.1 Serology of Delta virus infection

Radioimmunoassay and enzyme-linked immunosorbent assay (ELISA) (see Section 6.9) kits for detection of the Delta antigen (HDAg) and its corresponding IgM- and IgG-class antibodies are now commercially available and a molecular hybridization method for detection of the Delta virus RNA genome in serum has been developed [6]. These serological markers must be measured in conjunction with, and the findings interpreted in relation to, the various markers of HBV infection. It is important to note that the Delta virus interferes with HBV replication, leading to a transient fall in HBsAg titres and often a delay in appearance, or diminution in titres, of other HBV serum markers. In addition, Delta hepatitis is almost always accompanied by seroconversion from HBeAg to anti-HBe (section 5.3.2).

In *co-infection*, patients who have an uncomplicated acute Delta hepatitis typically do not develop a Delta viraemia (i.e. HDAg is not detected in the serum). HBsAg in serum follows the usual pattern seen in uncomplicated acute HBV hepatitis, with titres rising to a peak during the acute phase and falling during recovery (Fig. 5.6). At about the peak of HBsAg, IgM-anti-HDAg antibodies begin to appear in the serum accompanied by high-titre IgM-anti-HBc. The IgM-anti-HDAg rises in titre during the late acute phase then falls fairly rapidly, to be followed by a switch to the secondary (IgG) anti-HDAg response which often coincides with the appearance of anti-HBs. Once it appears, IgG-anti-HDAg may persist for years but, not infrequently, there is a delay in its appearance and this leaves a "window" between the IgM and IgG anti-HDAg responses during which there is no serological evidence of Delta infection. For this reason, it is customary to test several blood samples taken at intervals during and after the acute phase.

In *fulminant hepatitis* related to Delta co-infection, there is a transient Delta-antigenaemia but it is important to note that the serum must be treated with detergents to release HDAg from its HBsAg coat before it can be detected. The antigenaemia is followed by early seroconversion to IgM- and IgG-anti-HDAg, both classes of antibodies often appearing together and in conjunction with high-titre IgM-anti-HBc.

In HBV carriers who acquire Delta as a *super-infection*, HDAg appears in the serum at the onset of the acute Delta-induced hepatitis and is usually preceded by a decline in titres of HBsAg, which continue to decline until the Delta disappears (Fig. 5.7). Typically, these patients are *seronegative* for IgM-anti-HBc or have only low titres of this antibody. As Delta-antigenaemia wanes, both IgM- and IgG-anti-HDAg antibodies appear. Thereafter, the sequence of serological events depends on the clinical outcome. If the patient has an uncomplicated acute Delta hepatitis, IgM-anti-HDAg will disappear within a few months after recovery and persistence of IgG-anti-HDAg will be the only lasting evidence of the infection. However, the majority of super-infected individuals seem to develop chronic Delta hepatitis. Serologically, this can be diagnosed by the persistence of both IgM- and IgG-anti-HDAg antibodies in the serum (Fig. 5.7) and is very often associated with on-going liver damage as evidenced by persistently elevated serum aminotransferases and a histological picture of chronic active hepatitis. In these patients, titres of HBsAg tend to remain low.

The diagnosis of Delta infection can be difficult. Because the virus suppresses HBV replication and because of the "window" that

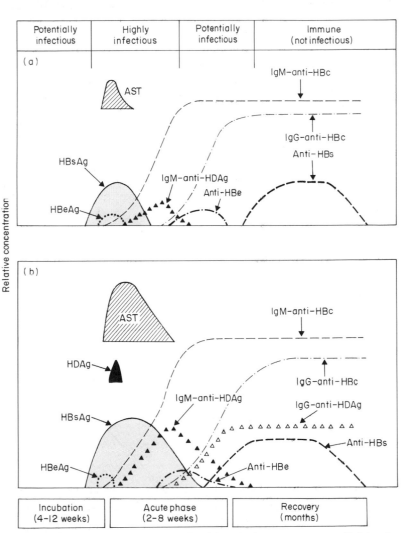

FIG 5.6. Serological events in (a) mild and (b) severe acute Delta virus co-infection.

sometimes occurs between the disappearance of IgM- and the appearance of IgG-anti-HDAg, a misdiagnosis of NANB hepatitis in a previously unsuspected carrier of HBV is possible. In addition, there is evidence that Delta stimulates the production of a variety of autoantibodies [7] and this could lead to a misdiagnosis of autoimmune chronic active hepatitis (see Chapter 6).

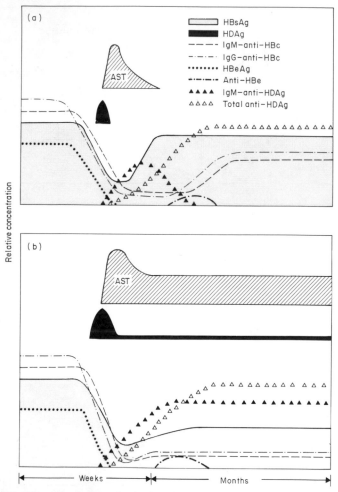

FIG 5.7. Typical serological events in (a) acute and (b) chronic Delta virus superinfection.

5.5 Non-A, non-B hepatitis viruses

Non-A, non-B (NANB) viral infections are now the most important cause of hepatitis following parenteral exposure to blood products and may also account for up to 25% of non-parenterally transmitted cases of presumed viral hepatitis. Precise knowledge of NANB hepatitis is sparse but is accumulating rapidly and it is likely that tests for the responsible agent(s) will soon be developed.

At the present time, clinical and epidemiological evidence suggests that there may be as many as four NANB viruses. Two of these seem to be transmitted enterically (faecal/oral route) and account for sporadic and epidemic outbreaks of NANB hepatitis. Like hepatitis A, these illnesses are usually self-limiting and chronic infections do not seem to occur. A third virus is responsible for transfusion-associated and other parenterally-transmitted outbreaks of NANB hepatitis and either this or a fourth virus accounts for other sporadic cases where no obvious source of infection can be identified, but where horizontal transmission through close contact appears to be important. Vertical (maternal/foetal) transmission also seems to occur [8].

In contrast to enteric NANB, parenterally-transmitted NANB is associated with a high rate of progression to chronic liver disease. Up to 60% of patients with acute post-transfusion NANB may develop chronic active hepatitis (with or without cirrhosis) [9, 10]. Since this can be confused with other forms of chronic hepatitis for which specific therapy is available (see Chapter 6), accurate diagnosis of chronic NANB hepatitis is exceedingly important.

However, at present, acute or chronic NANB hepatitis can only be diagnosed by exclusion of all other possible causes of the illness. HAV and HBV, as well as other viruses (see below) that can cause a hepatitic illness, must be excluded by appropriate serology. In chronic NANB, clinical, biochemical and histological investigations must be performed to exclude disorders such as haemochromatosis, Wilson's disease and other metabolic diseases affecting the liver (see Chapter 11). Screening for autoantibodies (Chapter 6) can be very useful, for these are rarely found in either acute or chronic NANB hepatitis and, when they do occur, are almost always at low titres [11]. In particular, patients with NANB are very rarely seropositive for anti-LSP or anti-ASGP-R antibodies (Chapter 6) and this distinguishes them from patients with hepatitis A or B infections and those with autoimmune chronic liver disease.

5.6 Other viral infections of the liver

There is a wide range of viruses (Table 5.1) capable of causing hepatitic illnesses that mimic those due to the hepatitis viruses (HAV, HBV and NANB) but, unlike HBV and NANB, progression to chronic liver disease is rare. In Europe and North America, the most important are the Epstein—Barr virus (infectious mononucleosis) and cytomegalovirus. The Arboviruses and Arenaviruses are of considerable importance in those parts of the world where they are endemic, but must also be considered if the patient has recently travelled to any of these territories. Other infections, such as those due to the coxsackie, echo, rubella, herpes simplex and varicella zoster viruses, because of their clinical features, generally do not present a major diagnostic problem but must be borne in mind.

Hepatitic symptoms, with elevated serum aminotransferase and/or bilirubin concentrations, due to Epstein—Barr virus (EBV) or cytomegalovirus (CMV) infections are probably more common in children than in adults. Up to 10% of patients with primary EBV infections will be jaundiced and 75% will have raised serum aminotransferases. CMV can be acquired *in utero* and will present as neonatal hepatitis, but in older children infections are often asymptomatic despite abnormalities in biochemical liver function tests (LFTs). Adults most at risk are those on immunosuppressive therapy (e.g. organ-transplant recipients) and persons receiving massive blood transfusions—about 10% of whom may be expected to develop CMV-related hepatitis, which may be severe. Herpes simplex infections in the newborn can cause severe (often fatal) liver damage and there have been occasional reports of a similar outcome in adults, especially during pregnancy. Severe varicella-related hepatitis has been reported in adults receiving immunosuppressive therapy.

Adenoviruses rarely cause hepatitis but there have been occasional outbreaks of hepatitic illnesses attributed to this group. The incidence of hepatitis associated with Arbo-, Arena-, Entero- and Marburg/Ebola viruses ranges from very frequent (Yellow Fever) to only occasional (Coxsackie) and from very severe to asymptomatic. The laboratory findings in Arbo-, Arena- and Marburg/Ebola infections are typical of acute hepatitis, with elevated serum aminotransferases (with or without jaundice), coagulation abnormalities and often evidence of renal dysfunction (oliguria, proteinuria). Up to 75% of neonates who acquire Rubella infections *in utero* will have some LFT abnormalities. These may be mild but more often are quite severe and

TABLE 5.1. Some viruses, other than the A, B and NANB viruses, that are capable of causing hepatitis in man.

Adenoviruses
   Various (rarely)
	Enteroviruses
	   Coxsackie A and B
	   Other enteroviruses

Arboviruses
   Dengue fever
   Kayasanur forest disease
   Rift Valley fever
   Yellow fever
	Herpes viruses
	   Cytomegalovirus
	   Epstein–Barr virus
	   Herpes simplex
	   Varicella zoster

Arenaviruses
   Argentinian haemorrhagic fever
   Bolivian haemorrhagic fever
   Lassa fever
	Marburg (green monkey)
	   and Ebola viruses
	Rubella and Rubeola

are an important consideration in the differential diagnosis of neonatal hepatitis (see Chapters 2 and 11).

Specific serological and/or biological tests for these viral infections exist and are available in many routine virology laboratories. A detailed discussion of these tests is beyond the scope of this book and the reader is referred to standard virology texts for further information.

5.7   Interpretation of laboratory tests

As a matter of routine, any patient with signs or symptoms of a hepatic illness should be screened for IgM-anti-HAV and for HBsAg. If these tests prove negative and a viral aetiology is still suspected, then the patient should be screened for other agents (particularly EBV and CMV; Section 5.7.4) and for IgM-anti-HBc (Section 5.3.2). Tests for Delta-virus infection are usually performed only when there is evidence of HBV infection (bearing in mind the "core window" phenomenon; Section 5.3.3).

With regard to routine tests for hepatitis viral markers, there are two important technical points to note.

(i) Whereas kits for measuring specific IgM-class antibodies against the various viral antigens are available, for technical reasons it has been difficult to develop routine methods for detecting the corresponding IgG-class antibodies on their own. Thus, the practice is to measure the total (IgM + IgG) antibody activity against the particular viral antigen and to compare this with the test result for the specific IgM antibody. If the latter is negative, it is assumed that the total activity is due to the IgG antibody.

(ii) Until recently, available kits were relatively insensitive and were capable of detecting many of the viral markers only when these were present at high levels in serum. The new generation of tests that are currently appearing are very much more sensitive and discrimination between high and low titres of certain markers is becoming clinically significant.

5.7.1 HAV markers

Because the viraemia is short-lived, it is not customary to test the

TABLE 5.2.   Interpretation of some typical results of tests for HAV infection

		Result			
	Test	1	2	3	4
A	*Total* anti-HAV	−	+	+	+
B	IgM-anti-HAV			+	−

Result	Interpretation	Comments
1	No recent exposure to HAV. Probably never exposed	Not immune to HAV
2	Recent infection with HAV *or* previous exposure to HAV	Might be infectious. Do test B
3	Recent/current infection with HAV	Potentially infectious. Repeat B in 2–4 weeks
4	Previous exposure to HAV	Immune to HAV. Not infectious

blood for hepatitis A antigen. The usual practice is to test for the *antibodies* induced by the virus and ELISA and RIA kits are available from commercial sources for detection of total and specific IgM-anti-HAV antibodies in serum. Although it is possible to titrate the antibodies, most laboratories report results simply as positive or negative, or semiquantitatively (i.e. weakly or strongly positive). This is adequate for most practical purposes, because the presence of IgM-anti-HAV indicates a recent infection and its disappearance accompanies recovery (Table 5.2).

Patients who are IgM-anti-HAV seropositive should be considered to be potentially capable of passing on the infection. Very rarely, IgM-anti-HAV may be detected in a person who has received a second exposure after a previous infection has rendered them immune. Such persons are likely to be asymptomatic and probably represent a low infectious risk but it is advisable to be cautious. In subjects who are negative for IgM-anti-HAV, seropositivity for total anti-HAV can be presumed to be due to the IgG antibody and, therefore, to reflect immunity to the virus following a previous infection.

5.7.2 HBV markers

The usual screening test for HBV infection involves the measurement of HBsAg in serum. As a general rule, a negative result is regarded as indicative of no current infection and is not further investigated. However, if there is reason to suspect a viral aetiology for the patient's symptoms or if the subject is a known contact of an HBV carrier, it may be worthwhile to carry out additional tests (Table 5.3) and to repeat these at intervals.

A positive HBsAg test, on its own, indicates only that the subject is currently infected with HBV and gives no information as to whether this is an acute or chronic infection. At the very least, HBsAg-positive subjects should be further tested for HBeAg and for anti-HBe, to establish their infectivity status, and should be re-tested for these markers and for anti-HBs at weekly or fortnightly intervals initially to determine whether the infection is acute or chronic.

Patients who are seropositive for HBeAg are highly infectious. Seroconversion to anti-HBe (Section 5.3.2) usually signals resolution of the infection, but this should be interpreted with caution, for active HBV (HBV-DNA positive) and concurrent Delta virus infections have been documented in anti-HBe-positive subjects (particularly in the Mediterranean areas and the Far East) [12]. If facilities are available,

TABLE 5.3. Interpretation of some commonly encountered results of tests for HBV infection

	Test	Result										
		1	2	3	4	5	6	7	8	9	10	11
A	HBsAg	−	−	−	−	−	−	−	+	+	+	+
B	HBeAg			−	−	−	−	−		+	+	−
C	Anti-HBs		−	−	−	−	+	+		−	−	−
D	Anti-HBe			−	−	+	−	−				
E	Total anti-HBc		−	+	+	+	+	−		−	+	+
F	IgM anti-HBc (high titre)		−	−	+	+	−	−		−	+	+

Result	Interpretation	Comments
1	No current HBV infection	If in doubt, do tests C, E and F
2	No current or previous HBV infection	Not immune
3	Previous (historic) exposure to HBV	May no longer be immune
4	Recent HBV infection, possibly still acute ("core window")	Still potentially highly infectious. Repeat A–E in 1–2 weeks
5	Recent HBV infection, early recovery phase	Potentially infectious but lower risk. Repeat A–E in 2–4 weeks
6	Previous HBV infection	Immune. Not infectious
7	Vaccinee, i.e. never previously exposed to full HBV infection	Immune. Not infectious
8	Current HBV infection, acute or chronic	Potentially highly infectious. Repeat A and do B–F[a]
9,10	Early acute HBV infection	Highly infectious. Repeat A–F weekly and test for Delta infection
11	Resolving acute or seroconverted chronic carrier	Potentially still infectious but lower risk. Repeat A–F weekly and test for Delta infection[a]

[a] If available, test for serum HBV-DNA or HBV-DNA polymerase.

the patient should be tested for serum HBV-DNA and/or HBV-DNA-polymerase (Section 5.3.1). Positive tests for either of these indicate that there is still active viral replication irrespective of the results of tests for the other HBV markers.

5.7.2.1 Acute hepatitis B

In uncomplicated acute hepatitis B, the timing of testing and variations between individuals in their response to the virus may be such that the classical sequence of serological markers may not be observed (Fig. 5.3). It is not uncommon for resolution of the illness, with disappearance of HBsAg and appearance of anti-HBs, to occur without HBeAg or anti-HBe ever having been detected. Generally, in acute hepatitis B the risk of transmitting the infection is considered to be low once HBeAg has disappeared. Where there is doubt, however, the patient should probably be considered to be potentially infectious until anti-HBs appears in the serum or, if that event is missed, until the disappearance of IgM-anti-HBc.

Rapidly declining titres of HBsAg with seroconversion to anti-HBe are typical findings in acute HBV infections that are resolving, but may also be seen in chronic HBV carriers with Delta virus super-infections (Section 5.4.1). If, despite declining HBsAg titres, there is persistence or worsening of symptoms and/or serum biochemical parameters, evidence of possible concurrent Delta or other virus infection should be sought (Sections 5.7.3 and 5.7.4) and non-viral causes of chronic liver disease should be excluded (see Chapters 6, and 9–12).

5.7.2.2 Chronic hepatitis B

When HBsAg persists in the serum for more than six months, the patient is considered to be a chronic carrier. It is now recognized that few such individuals are truly "healthy" and that most will have some changes in the liver, ranging from chronic persistent hepatitis (CPH) to florid chronic active hepatitis (CAH). The majority of these patients (including many with severe CAH) are asymptomatic or have only mild and relatively non-specific symptoms and may remain in this state for several years before their condition becomes clinically apparent (usually as a result of complications arising from advanced cirrhosis).

Biochemical LFTs are a little more helpful than clinical symptoms for identifying those carriers with more than minimal on-going hepatic injury, but even patients with severe CAH frequently have only modestly elevated (< two- to three-fold) serum aminotransferase activities and these tend to fluctuate, often becoming normal for a time before rising again. Perhaps more importantly, once an individual is known to be a carrier it is easy to attribute any abnormalities to the chronic HBV infection when, in fact, these may be due to other causes. Thus, it is essential to exclude Delta and other virus infections (Sections 5.7.3 and 5.7.4) as well as other causes of chronic liver disease (Chapters 6, and 9–12).

Tests for the full range of HBV markers should be performed at regular intervals to monitor the progress of the infection and to establish whether or not the patient is infectious (see Fig. 5.5). In the absence of a liver biopsy and with (the usual) equivocal biochemical LFT results, there are some serological tests that can be used as indicators of underlying hepatic injury. Thus, the presence of HBV-DNA or anti-HDAg in serum is almost always associated with on-going liver damage. Also, in our experience, the finding of high titres of anti-LSP and/or anti-ASGP-R autoantibodies (Chapter 6) in the sera of chronic HBV carriers always indicates severe liver damage (CAH), regardless of the severity of the serum biochemical abnormalities, but tests for these autoantibodies are not yet widely available.

5.7.3   HDV markers

Because Delta viraemia is usually of very short duration, tests for serum HDAg (Section 5.4.1) are often negative and for most practical purposes measurement of IgM-anti-HDAg and total anti-HDAg activity will suffice for investigating Delta-virus infections. These tests must be interpreted in relation to the results of concurrent tests for HBV serum markers (Table 5.4). In HBsAg-positive subjects, the absence of anti-HDAg indicates no previous exposure to the Delta virus and such patients (including "healthy carriers") must be considered at high risk of Delta-virus infection. In Europe and North America where Delta infection is at present mainly confined to certain high-risk groups (Section 5.4), testing for anti-HDAg can be a useful guide to the aetiology of the HBV infection, for finding anti-HDAg in serum together with IgM-anti-HBc is strongly suggestive of intravenous-drug abuse (which is usually denied initially).

In patients with acute hepatitis B whose illness follows a protracted or biphasic course despite apparent resolution on the basis of HBV

TABLE 5.4. Interpretation of some typical results of serological tests for Delta virus infection

	Test				Result			
		1	2	3	4	5	6	7
A	HDAg	−	−	+	−	+	−	±
B	Total anti-HDAg	−	+/−	±	+	+	+	+ +
C	IgM anti-HDAg	−	+	+	+/−	+	−	+ +
D	HBsAg	+	+	+	−	+	+	+
E	HBeAg	+/−	−	+/−	−	−/+	−	−/+
F	Anti-HBs	−	−	−	+	−	−	−
G	Anti-HBe	−/+	+/−	−/+	+/−	+/−	+/−	+/−
H	Total anti-HBc	+	+	+	+	−/±	+	±
I	IgM anti-HBc (high titre)	−/+	+	+ +	+	−/±	±	±

Result	Interpretation	Comments
1	No current or previous exposure to Delta virus	Susceptible to Delta infection. If in doubt, repeat B and C weekly for several weeks
2	Acute Delta co-infection	Potentially highly infectious. Repeat B–I weekly
3	Early severe acute Delta co-infection	Highly infectious. Repeat B–I weekly
4	Resolved acute Delta co-infection	Immune to Delta and to HBV. Not infectious
5	Early acute Delta super-infection	Highly infectious. Repeat B–I weekly
6	Resolved acute Delta super-infection	Immune to Delta. Still potentially infectious for HBV but lower risk
7	Chronic Delta infection	Highly infectious for Delta and probably also for HBV

serology (i.e. declining HBsAg titres and/or HBeAg/anti-HBe sero-conversion), Delta co-infection (Section 5.4) should be suspected. In this situation, the most useful serum marker is probably the IgM-anti-HDAg. In mild acute Delta hepatitis, this may be the only marker detected (Fig. 5.6a), but its appearance may be so transient that it is missed. In more severe Delta co-infections, it will usually be possible to detect IgM-anti-HDAg (Fig. 5.6b) but the timing of testing will be important, otherwise the results will be of historic interest only.

In chronic HBV carriers, unexpected acute hepatitic episodes or sudden declines in HBsAg titres raise the suspicion of Delta super-infection (Section 5.4). Such patients should be carefully monitored for progression to *chronic* Delta infection, which is associated with a poor prognosis. This can be documented by the persistence of IgM-anti-HDAg and sometimes also of low titres of HDAg in the serum (Fig. 5.7b).

5.7.4 Non-A, non-B and other viral infections

The difficulties relating to the diagnosis of NANB infections have been noted above (Section 5.5). At the outset, it is presumed that the patient will have been tested for IgM-anti-HAV and for HBsAg and found to be seronegative for both these markers. The next step should be to exclude occult HBV infection by testing for IgM-anti-HBc. Testing for total anti-HBc is of little value in this situation, because a positive result might be due to only IgG-anti-HBc from a previous HBV infection that is irrelevant in the present context.

If the patient is found to be IgM-anti-HBc seronegative, other viral infections (Section 5.6), particularly EBV and CMV, must be excluded and it may also be considered appropriate to screen for non-viral microbial infections (Chapter 12). Evidence for an underlying meta-bolic disease involving the liver (Chapter 11), of drug- or other chemically-induced liver damage (Chapter 9) and of excessive alcohol consumption (Chapter 10) must also be sought.

Finally, at some stage in this process, a full autoantibody screen (Chapter 6) should be requested to exclude an autoimmune aetiology. However, the absence of the standard non-organ-specific auto-antibodies (ANA, SMA, etc.) should be interpreted with caution, because it is becoming apparent that there are patients with steroid-responsive (presumed autoimmune) chronic active hepatitis who are seronegative for these autoantibodies. It has been found that such patients are almost always seropositive for anti-LSP and/or anti-

ASGP-R antibodies (Chapter 6) and this distinguishes them from patients with acute or chronic NANB hepatitis, who only very rarely have either of these liver autoantibodies.

5.8 Monitoring of hepatitis B virus vaccinees

The availability of vaccines against HBV infection is still too recent to establish firm criteria for monitoring response, predicting efficacy of protection, or deciding on whether (and, if so, when) booster doses should be given. However, a number of guidelines are emerging.

The current practice is to test vaccinees for serum anti-HBs at between one and three months after the final dose of a course of the vaccine. In most populations that have been studied, the resulting anti-HBs levels have been found to fall into one of three groups: (i) *high* responders (anti-HBs levels of $> 1000\,IU\,l^{-1}$); (ii) *hypo*-responders (levels of $10-100\,IU\,l^{-1}$); and (iii) *non*-responders (levels of $< 10\,IU\,l^{-1}$).

The degree of protection seems to be directly related to the anti-HBs response elicited by the vaccine. Booster doses given (e.g. at 12 and 18 months) improve anti-HBs levels in about half of the *hypo*- and *non*-responders, but seldom to the levels seen in high responders. Frequent monitoring of anti-HBs levels in vaccinees is costly and is generally considered unnecessary because the level at the end of the initial course establishes the subject's response to the particular vaccine, but it is probably worthwhile to re-test individuals receiving booster doses to establish whether their anti-HBs levels have risen above the currently recommended minimum of $50\,IU\,l^{-1}$. However, *hypo*- and *non*-responders and those who fail to complete the recommended course of vaccination *should be considered not to be fully protected* even if their levels rise above $50\,IU\,l^{-1}$ after a booster dose. In these subjects, the practice is to err on the side of caution and to offer passive immunoprophylaxis following a definite exposure to HBV. Current recommendations are that *high* responders should receive booster doses after five years.

New vaccines are appearing and others will follow shortly. Some of these include the pre-S components of HBV coat protein (Section 5.3.1) and tests for anti-pre-S and/or anti-pHSAr are likely to be recommended for monitoring individuals receiving these vaccines.

References

1. Lever AML. J Hepatol 1987; 4: 399.
2. Coursaget P et al. Lancet 1987; ii: 1354.
3. MacKay P et al. J Med Virol 1981; 8: 237.
4. Neurath AP et al. Nature 1985; 315: 154.
5. Buitrago B et al. Hepatology 1986; 6: 1292.
6. Smedile A et al. Hepatology 1986; 6: 1297.
7. Crivelli O et al. Cln Exp Immunol 1983; 54: 232.
8. Tong MJ et al. Gastroenterology 1981; 80: 999.
9. Koretz RL et al. Gastroenterology 1980; 79: 893.
10. Gealdi G et al. Gut 1982; 23: 270.
11. Mackay IR et al. Clin Exp Immunol 1985; 61: 39.
12. Lock ASF et al. Gut 1984; 25: 1283.

Suggested further reading

Alter HJ, Hepatitis. Sem Liver Dis 1986; 6: 1—95.
Bianchi L. The immunopathology of acute type B hepatitis. Springer Sem Immunopathol 1981; 3: 421—438.
Fagan EA (1988). Practical aspects of hepatitis B vaccination. Gastroenterol Pract 1988; June/July: 21—26.
Fagan E, Vergani D and Williams R. Conference: Delta hepatitis. Lancet 1987; ii: 1322—1323.
Fagan EA and Williams R. Progress report: Serological responses to HBV infection. Gut 1986; 27: 858—867.
Hoofnagle JH, Shafritz DA and Popper H. Chronic type B hepatitis and the "healthy" HBsAg carrier state. Hepatology 1987; 7: 758—763.
Lever AML. Mechanisms of virally induced liver damage. J Hepatol 1987; 4: 399—403.
Levy GA and Chisari FV. The immunopathogenesis of chronic HBV-induced liver disease. Springer Sem Immunopathol 1981; 3: 439—459.
Lindsay KL, Nizze JA, Koretz R and Gitnick G. Diagnostic usefulness of testing for anti-HBc IgM in acute hepatitis B. Hepatology 1986; 6: 1325—1328.
MacSween RNM. Pathology of viral hepatitis and its sequelae. Clinics Gastroenterology 1980; 9: 23—32.
Paz Moa, Brenes F, Karayiannis P et al. Chronic hepatitis B virus infection. Viral replication and patterns of inflammatory activity: Serological, clinical and histological correlations. J Hepatol 1986; 3: 371—377.
Rakela J, Taswell HF and Ludwig J. Chronic non-A, non-B hepatitis. In:

Chronic Active Hepatitis — The Mayo Clinic Experience. New York: Marcel Dekker, 1986, Chapter 10.

Rizetto M and Verme G. Delta hepatitis — present status. J Hepatol 1985; 1: 187–193.

Schalm SW, Davis GL and Shiels MT. Chronic active hepatitis type B. In: Chronic Active Hepatitis — The Mayo Clinic Experience. New York: Marcel Dekker, 1986, Chapter 9.

Shearman DJC and Finlayson NDC. Diseases of the Gastrointestinal Tract and Liver. Edinburgh: Churchill Livingstone, 1982, Chapter 25.

Sherlock S and Thomas HC. Conference report: Delta virus hepatitis. J Hepatol 1985; 3: 419–423.

Theilmann L. Pfaff E, Kommerell B. *et al*. Detection of hepatitis B virus core gene products in sera and liver of HBV-infected individuals. J Hepatol 1989; 8: 77–85.

Verme G, Bonino F and Rizetto M. (Eds). Viral Hepatitis and Delta Infection. Progress in Clinical and Biological Research, Vol. 143. New York: Alan R. Liss, 1983.

6

Immunology

6.1 Introduction

For all practical purposes, apart from screening for lupus erythematosus (LE) cells (see below), immunological investigations in liver
disease are primarily concerned with serology. Notwithstanding the
interesting association of an assortment of histocompatibility antigens
with autoimmune chronic active hepatitis (AI-CAH), primary sclerosing cholangitis (PSC), some forms of alcoholic liver disease (ALD)
and haemochromatosis, investigations of these and other cellular
aspects of the immune system in various liver disorders (although of
considerable research interest) are technically too cumbersome for
routine clinical use at the present time. Thus, the main immunological
investigations are concerned with the measurement of serum immunoglobulins and autoantibodies. Detection of circulating immune complexes, investigations of abnormalities of complement metabolism
and measurement of acute-phase reactants in serum are also performed routinely but less frequently.

These investigations are of value principally in the differential
diagnosis of chronic liver disease, a term that encompasses a spectrum
of disorders including AI-CAH, PSC, ALD (Chapter 10) and haemochromatosis (Chapter 11) as well as: primary biliary cirrhosis (PBC),
chronic infection with hepatitis-B virus (HBV) or the non-A, non-B
(NANB) viruses (Chapter 5), drug-induced liver damage (Chapter 9),
Wilson's disease and α_1-antitrypsin deficiency (Chapter 11) and a wide
range of microbial infections other than the hepatitis viruses (Chapter
12). Most of these disorders can present as chronic active hepatitis
(CAH) and accurate diagnosis is essential, because specific therapy is
available for some conditions (e.g. Wilson's disease, haemochromatosis), while corticosteroid therapy, which is of benefit in AI-CAH, may
be of questionable value or even contraindicated in others (e.g. HBV-
or NANB-CAH, PBC).

6.2 LE cells

The lupus erythematosus (LE)-cell phenomenon was first described by Hargreaves in 1948 in blood smears from patients with systemic lupus (SLE). The LE cell is a phagocytic leucocyte containing a large, Feulgen-positive, cytoplasmic inclusion comprising a cell nucleus (with adherent 7S-IgG and complement components) that has been extruded from a damaged lymphocyte and engulfed by the phagocyte. LE cells are normally associated with the presence of anti-dsDNA antibodies (Section 6.4.1) in the patient's serum and it is thought that these constitute the 7S-IgG attached to the extruded lymphocyte nucleus, resulting in an immune complex and consequent activation of complement.

6.3 Serum immunoglobulins

Hyperglobulinaemia is a common finding in liver disease (particularly in the chronic liver disorders) and is usually due to an increase in the gamma-globulin fraction, which includes the serum immuno-globulins. At least part of the increase may be a consequence of enhanced antigenic stimulation of the immune system as a result of inadequate phagocytic elimination by the liver of gut-derived anti-gens, due to porto–systemic shunting (Section 1.3.1). Often, however, the hyperglobulinaemia is indicative of an underlying inflammatory process involving the liver.

The quantitative estimation of specific immunoglobulin classes (IgG, IgA, IgM) can be quite useful in diagnosis because some liver disorders are associated with preferential increases in serum levels of IgG, IgA and/or IgM, even when total globulin concentrations are within the normal range (Section 6.8.2).

Measurements of serum immunoglobulin classes may be made using a variety of techniques (see Section 6.9), including immunodiffusion, immuno-electrophoresis, enzyme-linked immunosorbent assay (ELISA), radioim-munoassay (RIA) or (increasingly) nephelometry, by using commercially available class-specific anti-immunoglobulin antisera.

6.4 Autoantibodies

Circulating autoantibodies are immunoglobulins (usually IgG, but also IgM and occasionally IgA) that recognize and bind to normal ("self") constituents of tissues. They are generally classified as *organ-specific* or *non-organ-specific* according to the tissue distribution of the "self" antigens with which they react. Thus, the former react with antigens that are present in only one tissue (or, at most, a very limited number of tissues), whereas the target antigens of non-organ-specific autoantibodies (e.g. ANA, SMA, AMA, see below) have a broad tissue distribution.

6.4.1 Antinuclear antibodies

The term antinuclear antibody (ANA) describes a spectrum of auto-antibodies that react with a variety of nuclear antigens, many of which have been characterized (Table 6.1). Screening for ANAs is usually performed by indirect immunofluorescence (IF) on rodent tissue sections or other appropriate substrates (Section 6.9.2). Some specialist laboratories will provide an "ANA profile", detailing the antigenic specificities of the ANA detected by routine IF, but so far this has been of value mainly in the connective-tissue disorders and the relevance (if any) of various specificities of ANA to particular liver diseases is not yet fully understood.

Depending on the substrate employed, four distinct patterns of IF staining are recognized: (i) *homogeneous*, diffuse staining over the whole nucleus; (ii) *speckled*, a particulate pattern which may be fine and uniform or granular and clumpy; (iii) *peripheral*, outlining the rim of the nucleus; and (iv) *nucleolar*. The pattern of staining can provide a clue to the target antigen involved as well as to the disease with which the particular ANA is associated. Thus, the homogeneous pattern is typical of that given by ANAs in the sera of patients with systemic lupus erythematosus (SLE), the uniform speckled pattern is characteristic of the anti-centromere antibody associated with progressive systemic sclerosis (scleroderma) and, more particularly, with the *CREST* syndrome (calcinosis, Raynaud's phenomenon, oesophageal dysmotility, sclerodactyly and telangiectasia), while the clumpy speckled pattern is seen with (but not exclusive to) antibodies against the non-histone nucleoproteins Sm and La (SS-B) which are found, respectively, in SLE and in Sjogren's syndrome.

TABLE 6.1 Some sub-specificities of ANAs and their more common disease associations[a]

Antibody	Disease associations
ANA (homogeneous IF pattern)	SLE, AI-CAH, PSC, PBC, drug-induced lupus (also, older healthy subjects)
Anti-dsDNA By Farr assay	SLE, AI-CAH, HBV-CAH, AVH, ALD, PBC
By other RIAs or by *Crithidia luciliae* IF	SLE only
Anti-centromere	Scleroderma, CREST syndrome, PBC
Anti-Ro(SSA) and anti-La(SSB)	Primary Sjogren's syndrome, SLE, congenital heart block, PBC
Anti-histone	Drug-induced lupus, SLE
Anti-Sm	SLE
Anti-nRNP	Mixed connective-tissue disease (high titres). Other connective-tissue disorders (low titres)
Anti-RANA	Rheumatoid arthritis

[a] See text for explanation of abbreviations.

Techniques for ANA screening differ between laboratories and clinical interpretation of results depends on a knowledge of precisely what method has been used. For example, ANAs that react with the phosphoribosyl backbone of the DNA helix in double-stranded DNA (dsDNA) are conventionally detected by the Farr assay (Section 6.9.5) but may be determined by other RIAs, by haemagglutination (Section 6.9.6) or by ELISA (Section 6.9.3), using purified dsDNA from which all traces of single-stranded DNA have been removed. They are also detected by IF, using as substrate the protozoan *Crithidia luciliae* (Section 6.9.2), which has a modified mitochondrion (the kinetoplast) thought to contain only dsDNA. When determined by the Farr assay, high titres of anti-dsDNA antibodies can be found frequently in the sera of patients with SLE as well as in patients with acute viral hepatitis, idiopathic or HBV-related CAH, alcoholic liver disease, or primary biliary cirrhosis [1], irrespective of whether the patients are seropositive for ANA by IF on tissue sections. However, if the same sera are tested by other RIAs or by the *Crithidia luciliae* method, usually only those from SLE patients will yield a positive result.

Among the other ANA specificities, the antihistone activity associated with drug-induced lupus (Table 6.1) is worth noting. Anti-histone antibodies also occur in about 30% of SLE patients but are directed at a different class of histones to that recognized by ANA in drug-induced lupus. Some laboratories still offer testing for antibodies against "extractable nuclear antigen" (ENA). The latter comprises a group of nuclear antigens that can be extracted with buffered saline and "anti-ENA" is therefore of quite broad specificity. ANAs that recognize antigenic structures on the nucleotide bases of single-stranded DNA occur in such a wide range of conditions that they are of little diagnostic value.

6.4.2 Anti-smooth-muscle antibodies

Anti-smooth-muscle antibodies (SMA) reacting with a broad range of tissues were first described in the sera of patients with chronic liver disease but were subsequently found to occur at high frequency in acute viral hepatitis (AVH) as well as in a wide range of acute and chronic microbial and other conditions not necessarily involving the liver [2, 3]. In acute infections, the SMA tend to occur transiently and at relatively low titres and are usually predominantly of the IgM class. The highest titres are seen in patients with untreated AI-CAH, up to 85% of whom may be SMA-positive. In this condition the SMA are specific for the smooth-muscle protein F-actin, which distinguishes them from autoantibodies reacting with other muscle components in some other diseases.

SMA are routinely detected by indirect immunofluorescence using rodent tissue sections (Section 6.9.2). Most laboratories employ rat stomach and kidney as substrate, on which the SMA stain the gastric muscularis mucosae and the renal blood vessels as well as (to a lesser extent) the glomeruli and tubular epithelial cells. However, SMA will react with smooth-muscle fibres in almost any tissue, including intestinal epithelium, the microfilaments of hepatocytes and the membrane region of thyroid epithelial cells.

6.4.3 Anti-mitochondrial antibodies

Anti-mitochondrial antibodies (AMA) represent a broad group of autoantibodies that react with several different antigens in mitochondria and most sub-specificities of AMA are associated with particular diseases, including some disorders that do not always involve the liver (Table 6.2).

At least nine different specificities (M1–M9) of AMA are recognized, ranging from anti-cardiolipin (M1) to an antibody (M9) that reacts only with mitochondria in the liver. The M2-AMA is directed at a trypsin-sensitive antigen on the inner side of the mitochondrial membrane and is highly specific for PBC, while the M4-AMA (directed at a trypsin-insensitive outer mitochondrial membrane antigen) appears to identify those cases of PBC that overlap with AI-CAH and *vice versa*.

AMA are routinely detected by indirect IF (Section 6.9.2) on unfixed cryostat sections of rat kidney, liver and stomach. They give a characteristic staining of mitochondria in the distal renal tubular epithelial cells and also stain mitochondria in hepatocytes and gastric parietal cells. Several other techniques, including ID, RIA, ELISA, complement fixation and dot-immunobinding (Section 6.9), have been developed for AMA detection but these are used mainly by specialized laboratories. Experienced observers may be able to distinguish between some of the different AMAs according to the IF staining patterns but more precise techniques (RIA, ELISA, complement fixation) using the purified target antigens are usually required to discriminate between the various specificities.

TABLE 6.2 Disease associations of various AMAs

AMA specificity	Associated disorders
M1	Secondary syphilis
M2	Primary biliary cirrhosis
M3	Drug-induced pseudo-lupus syndrome
M4	"Overlap" cases of primary biliary cirrhosis and autoimmune CAH
M5	Some SLE patients
M6	Drug-induced hepatitis
M7	Various cardiomyopathies
M8	Primary biliary cirrhosis
M9	Primary biliary cirrhosis and some healthy subjects

6.4.4 Liver–kidney microsomal antibodies

Liver–kidney microsomal (LKM) autoantibodies were first characterized by Rizetto and co-workers in 1973 [4, 5]. These antibodies were originally described in the sera of a small number of patients with idiopathic CAH and very occasionally in other disorders. It was found that the target of the LKM is located in the microsomal membranes and recent studies have shown that there are at least two such autoantibodies, LKM-1 and LKM-2. Both are directed at the cytochrome P-450 complex in the smooth endoplasmic reticulum [6, 7], but it appears that they react with different P-450 isoenzymes. LKM-1 is associated with the sub-group of idiopathic (probably autoimmune) CAH and LKM-2 is found in patients with drug-induced hepatitis.

By IF, LKM antibodies give a fine granular staining of the cytoplasm of hepatocytes and a slightly more irregular pattern on a limited number of other tissues, mainly kidney, that requires an experienced eye to distinguish from the staining given by AMA (Section 6.4.3). However, LKM can be relatively easily distinguished from AMA during routine IF screening by the absence of staining on sections of stomach.

6.4.5 Liver-membrane antibody

Liver-membrane antibody (LMA) is directed at a liver-specific antigen located in the plasma membranes of hepatocytes [8]. The antibody is detected by indirect immunofluorescence (Section 6.9.2), using mechanically isolated non-viable hepatocytes on which it gives a smooth "linear" pattern of surface membrane staining that must be distinguished from a "granular" pattern given by sera (e.g. from patients with HBV infections or PBC) that contain immune complexes (Section 6.5). The fact that LMA does not react with enzymically isolated viable hepatocytes (in which the integrity of the plasma membrane has been preserved) is taken to indicate that the target antigen, LMAg, is not located on the outer surfaces of liver cells but is a submembranous component which is not normally exposed [9].

Several attempts have been made to develop other techniques (RIA, ELISA) or variations on the immunofluorescence method for detection of LMA, but all are subject to technical considerations that raise questions about the interpretation of the results (Section 6.8.4). In addition, the problem of how to detect the antibody in LMA-positive sera that also contain immune complexes has not yet been satisfactorily resolved. LMA seems to be primarily an IgG antibody, but there is some evidence that IgM- or IgA-class LMA may also exist.

6.4.6 Anti-LSP antibodies

Anti-LSP is the term used to describe a group of autoantibodies (as yet not fully defined) which react with antigens in a preparation from normal liver known as liver-specific membrane lipoprotein (LSP) [10]. This is a fairly crude but well-standardized preparation containing fragments of liver cell membranes, including hepatocellular plasma membranes. The antibodies are detected by radioimmunoassay or by ELISA (Section 6.9.5) but, in our experience [10], the latter method is prone to give false positive results.

Anti-LSP antibodies occur in a wide range of liver disorders in which there is some underlying immunopathology and, in the chronic liver diseases, is particularly associated with periportal inflammation and piecemeal necrosis. One of the constituent antigens in LSP, the asialoglycoprotein receptor protein (Section 6.4.7), has been identified but there is evidence to indicate that there are other important antigens in this preparation and that the antigenic targets of anti-LSP antibodies differ between the various liver disorders.

6.4.7 Anti-ASGP-R antibodies

Anti-ASGP-R autoantibodies are directed at the hepatic asialoglycoprotein receptor (ASGP-R) protein. This receptor was originally known as hepatic lectin (HL) [11], but the term has now largely fallen into disuse because of a tendency for confusion with other animal and plant lectins and will be avoided here. ASGP-R is involved in the endocytic removal of galactose-terminating desialylated serum glycoproteins. It is functionally and immunochemically specific to the liver and is expressed on the sinusoidal and basolateral surfaces of the plasma membrane. Perhaps not surprisingly, in view of the membrane content of LSP (see above), ASGP-R is a component of the LSP preparation. It comprises only about $0 \cdot 25\%$ of the total protein in LSP but it is highly immunogenic and thus represents a major antigenic constituent of the LSP preparation [12]. Autoantibodies against ASGP-R are detected by RIA (Section 6.9.5) and constitute part of the total anti-LSP activity in some anti-LSP positive sera in certain liver disorders (Section 6.8.4).

6.4.8   Anti-SLA antibody

Anti-SLA is an autoantibody that reacts with a soluble cytoplasmic antigen (SLA) which, although present at highest concentrations in the liver, can be found in a wide range of tissues and is thus not liver-specific [13]. The antibody is measured by RIA (Section 6.9.5). It cannot be detected by standard IF techniques. Anti-SLA seems to be distinct from other autoantibodies such as ANA, SMA, AMA, anti-LKM and LMA, because it has been found in sera that are negative for all of these. It also appears to be distinct from anti-LSP because its target antigen (SLA) is not a constituent of LSP preparations [13]

6.4.9   Hepatocyte membrane antibodies

Hepatocyte membrane antibodies (HMA) represent what appears to be a group of autoantibodies that react with antigens in liver cell plasma membranes. They are detected by indirect IF (Section 6.9.2) on rat liver sections that have been fixed in Bouin's solution (picric acid/formalin/acetic acid), on which they give a linear polygonal pattern of plasma membrane staining outlining the hepatocytes [14]. They cannot be detected when unfixed frozen tissue sections are used, which probably indicates that the target antigens are very soluble and are lost during the obligatory washing of the sections. An advantage of this, however, is that staining due to ANA and SMA (which would confuse) is abolished by Bouin's fixation. The target antigens of HMA are not yet known but some seem to be shared with LSP (Section 6.4.6) and/or with polymerized human serum albumin (pHSA), for HMA titres in some positive sera can be considerably reduced by prior absorption with LSP or pHSA.

6.5   Immune complexes and complement

Circulating immune complexes (CIC) are detectable by a variety of techniques, each with its own specificity and sensitivity [15]. CIC occur in a wide range of disorders including several autoimmune diseases (e.g. SLE, rheumatoid arthritis), numerous microbial infections (e.g. viral hepatitis, malaria, leprosy, infective endocarditis, onchocerciasis, Dengue fever) and many malignant conditions (e.g. leukaemia, most lymphomas, melanomas, and carcinomas of breast, lung, stomach and colon). They comprise antigens and antibodies in different ratios which determine the ultimate sizes of the complexes. The antigens may be normal tissue components (autoantigens), dietary immunogens, or of microbial origin, while the antibodies can be of any of the three immunoglobulin classes.

Interest in CIC derives from the fact that they may activate complement or physically congest capillaries (and stimulate release of vasoactive amines with consequent local tissue damage) as well as from the possibility that their constituent antibodies and/or antigens may be related to pathogenesis or that the complexes may modulate immune responses by direct effects on lymphocytes. Their presence is usually associated with vasculitis, arthritis, glomerulonephritis or skin lesions and, because some CIC precipitate on cooling and redissolve on rewarming (a characteristic of cryoglobulins) they may be involved in circulatory disorders such as Raynaud's phenomenon. CIC have been demonstrated in several liver diseases, mainly those in which the above extrahepatic complications are common, but their relevance (if any) to primary pathogenesis of the liver disorders is unclear [16].

In certain liver conditions (notably PBC), derangements of either the classical or alternate pathways of complement metabolism can be demonstrated [17, 18]. It seems likely that, in at least some of these conditions, the complement abnormalities may be related to the presence of CIC. The measurement of complement components is becoming more routine and the findings in patients with liver disease may prove useful in diagnosis and clinical management, but this is still under assessment.

6.6 Cryoglobulins

Cryoglobulins are serum proteins that precipitate on cooling and redissolve on rewarming. They are detected by allowing the blood sample at clot to 37°C and then leaving the separated serum to stand in a tube at 4°C for several days. Often, the presence of cryoglobulins will become evident after a few hours by the development of a flocculent precipitate in the tube and this can be confirmed by observing the disappearance of the precipitate upon rewarming the serum to 37°C and its reappearance when the sample is again placed at

4°C. Because some cryoproteins precipitate only very slowly, it is important to leave the serum sample for at least seven days at 4°C before declaring it cryoglobulin-negative. Fairly precise quantitative estimates of amounts of cryoglobulins in a serum sample can be made by removing the precipitate by centrifugation at 4°C, washing it and measuring the protein content by standard techniques.

Cryoglobulins are a relatively non-specific phenomenon, often related to circulating immune complexes and associated with a similar range of disorders (Section 6.5), but the relative ease with which they can be detected has led to their measurement perhaps more often than has been clinically necessary.

6.7 Acute-phase reactants

In most inflammatory conditions, infections, and where tissue damage has occurred (e.g. due to trauma), transient and selective increases in the concentrations of a wide range of serum proteins can be demonstrated (Table 6.3). These changes are part of what is known as the *acute-phase response*, hence acute-phase proteins. Many of these proteins can now be measured by using commercially available specific antisera with techniques such as ID, IEP, RIA, ELISA (Section 6.9) that can be performed in most routine laboratories.

The majority of the acute-phase proteins are synthesized by the liver (some exclusively so) but the stimuli that induce the acute-phase response are so diverse and the selective increases in the blood levels of the different proteins are so variable (even within a single disease entity) that, with certain notable exceptions (α_1-antitrypsin, pro-

TABLE 6.3   Plasma proteins that may be increased in concentration during the acute-phase response

α_1-acid glycoprotein (orosomucoid)	Fibrinogen
α_1-antitrypsin	Fibronectin
α_1-antichymotrypsin	Gc globulin
Ceruloplasmin	Haptoglobin
Complement components	Haemopexin
C-reactive protein	Prothrombin
Ferritin	Serum amyloid A protein

thrombin, ceruloplasmin, ferritin, for reasons unconnected with the acute-phase response), the routine estimation of these proteins has so far proved to be of little practical clinical value in liver disease.

6.8 Interpretation of immunological tests

The results of immunological tests need to be considered in the overall clinical context. In addition to the relevant signs and symptoms, account should be taken of the age and sex of the patient (immunological abnormalities are more common in females), travel to countries where certain microbial infections are endemic, recent blood transfusions or inoculations, drug and alcohol history and exposure to other potentially hepatotoxic agents (Chapter 9), and allergies and other co-existing disorders. Often, the interpretation will be quite straightforward because there are already grounds for suspecting chronic liver disease. It is not uncommon, however, for patients with quite severe chronic liver disease to have relatively mild symptoms and/or serum biochemical abnormalities and for their condition to be revealed by immunological tests. Also, occasionally, routine health screening will reveal an immunological abnormality which is the only evidence of a serious underlying condition (e.g. AMA in asymptomatic PBC; see Section 6.8.3).

6.8.1 LE cells

In liver disease, the presence of LE cells (Section 6.2) was used to classify those patients with CAH in whom the disorder was thought to be related to autoimmunity (AI-CAH). Subsequently, the definition of AI-CAH was broadened to include patients with idiopathic CAH whose sera contain ANA and/or SMA (Section 6.4), whether or not LE cells are present. Screening for LE cells has consequently diminished in importance, for they occur in less than 30% of patients fulfilling this wider definition of AI-CAH. In addition to their association with SLE and other connective-tissue disorders, LE cells are also found in some patients with HBV-CAH, mainly those who have circulating ANA.

6.8.2 Serum immunoglobulins

Elevations of the total globulin fraction of serum (Chapter 2) are often indicative of an underlying inflammatory process. At the very least, this should be confirmed by requesting the laboratory to perform an electrophoretic separation of the serum to determine whether the abnormality is related to an increase in the gamma-globulin fraction. Preferably, the specific classes (IgG, IgA, IgM) of the serum immunoglobulins should be measured and an autoantibody screen (Section 6.4) should be requested.

Increases in serum IgM and IgG, or all three classes together, often occur in microbial infections. The magnitude of these increases will depend on the individual, on the timing of presentation and on the stage, nature and severity of the infection. Levels may continue to rise for a time after presentation but should begin to return towards normal after the initial acute phase has passed and this can be

TABLE 6.4   Typical patterns of changes in the serum concentrations of IgG, IgA and IgM in some liver disorders

Liver disorder	IgG	IgA	IgM
Acute virus A or B hepatitis	↑ or ⬆ (transient)	N or ↑ (transient)	↑ or ⬆ (transient)
Acute NANB viral hepatitis and other microbial infections	N or ↑ (transient)	N	N or ↑ (transient)
Autoimmune CAH (untreated)	↑ or ⬆	N or ↑	N or ↑
HBV- and NANB-CAH	N or ↑	N	N or ↑
Primary biliary cirrhosis	N or ↑	N or ↑	↑ or ⬆
Alcoholic liver disease	N or ↑	↑ or ⬆	N
Haemochromatosis	N	N	N
Wilson's disease	N or ↑	N	N

N, normal; ↑, slightly increased (< two-fold); ⬆, markedly increased (> two-fold).

demonstrated by re-testing at intervals of a few days during the illness. In any event, when there is an increase in more than one immunoglobulin class, microbial infection (see Chapters 5 and 12) should always be considered as a possible cause of the abnormality (Table 6.4). Other causes not necessarily involving the liver include most of the connective tissue disorders and some of the gammopathies. Decreases in serum immunoglobulin classes are usually confined to certain immunodeficiency states and to the monoclonal gammopathies in which an increase in one class may be accompanied by decreases in the other two classes.

When microbial infections have been excluded, the finding of a selective increase in serum IgM levels to more than two or three times the normal upper limit in a patient with suspected liver disease is suggestive of primary biliary cirrhosis (PBC), particularly in a female over 30 years of age. However, this is not a prerequisite for a diagnosis of PBC, for many patients (especially asymptomatic cases [19]) do present with normal or near-normal IgM levels. Often, PBC patients will also have elevated serum concentrations of IgG (usually less than two-fold), but IgA levels tend to be normal or only slightly raised.

A preferential elevation in serum IgG is usually associated with CAH. The increase may be fairly modest (less than two-fold), especially in CAH due to hepatitis virus (HBV, NANB) infections, but in CAH of other aetiologies (Section 6.1) rises of three-fold or more are not uncommon and an increase in total serum globulin with specific elevation of serum IgG is part of the diagnostic criteria for AI-CAH. Selective increases in serum IgA concentrations are typically seen in alcoholic liver disease (Chapter 10).

The total serum globulin concentration can be used as a rough guide to responses to therapy in AI-CAH, but it is important to note that increases in the serum concentrations of individual immunoglobulin classes can occur in patients with normal total globulin levels. It is often worthwhile, therefore, to request a serum immunoglobulin profile regardless of the total globulin concentration. Also, immunosuppressive therapy can quite dramatically and preferentially reduce serum immunoglobulin concentrations. For example, in patients with AI-CAH who are receiving corticosteroids, it is not uncommon for the serum IgG level to return to normal before the biochemical LFTs. Thus, the serum immunoglobulin profile can be useful for monitoring early responses to therapy in these situations. However, the corollary, i.e. early *increases* in serum IgG heralding relapse when treatment is reduced or withdrawn, does not invariably apply.

123

6.8.3 ANA, SMA and AMA

Most routine laboratories will provide an autoantibody screen for antinuclear (ANA), anti-smooth-muscle (SMA) and anti-mitochondrial (AMA) antibodies. Since this will usually be done by IF on sections of kidney, liver and stomach (Section 6.4), the finding of gastric parietal cell antibodies may also be reported and many laboratories will routinely include additional tests for rheumatoid factor and anti-thyroid antibodies. The latter three are of little specific relevance to liver disease but can provide useful background information about possible co-existing autoimmune disorders.

It is important to recognize that, with the possible exception of AMA (Table 6.2), none of the non-organ-specific autoantibodies is unique to any liver disorder. In addition to their prevalence in non-hepatic autoimmune diseases, many of these antibodies occur quite frequently (albeit usually transiently) in a wide variety of acute or chronic microbial infections, including hepatitis A and B, cyto-megalovirus, mycoplasma, malaria, leprosy, and even in patients with plantar warts. Also, while titres of IgM- and/or IgG-class ANA and/or SMA up to 1 : 80 occur in less than 5% of healthy subjects under 40 years of age, the frequency rises to about 25% in those who are over 60 years. Conversely, it is becoming apparent that there is a group of patients with steroid-responsive chronic liver disease who are persistently ANA- and SMA-seronegative, but in whom the disease may have an autoimmune aetiology.

The interpretation of a positive or negative ANA or SMA result in the context of suspected liver disease is therefore by no means straightforward. Microbial infections and pre-existing autoimmune diseases that are normally associated with these autoantibodies must be excluded and, in patients with conditions such as rheumatoid arthritis, the possibility must be considered that the autoantibodies are a reflection of that disorder and that the liver abnormalities may be due to a condition (e.g. NANB hepatitis, haemochromatosis, Budd–Chiari or Gilbert's syndromes) that is unrelated to autoimmunity. Also, whether or not there is evidence of a co-existing disorder, it must be borne in mind that the titre of the autoantibody may not be abnormal for the age of the individual concerned.

When account has been taken of the above, the finding of ANA or SMA in a patient with suspected liver disease is usually taken to indicate that there is some immunopathological, probably auto-immune, disorder. The presence of either of these autoantibodies at titres of 1 : 40 or greater is considered by some clinicians to be part of

TABLE 6.5 Approximate frequencies of ANA, SMA and AMA in various disorders and in normal subjects

	ANA	SMA	AMA
Chronic active hepatitis			
Autoimmune (untreated)	VF	VF	Occ
HBV-related	Occ	Occ	R
NANB-CAH	R	R	R
Acute viral hepatitis			
Virus A or B	F (T)	VF (T)	R (T)
NANB viruses	R (T)	R (T)	O
Other microbial infections[a]	Occ (T)	Occ (T)	O
Primary biliary cirrhosis	F	F	I
Alcoholic liver disease	F	F	R
Primary sclerosing cholangitis	Var	Var	R
Wilson's disease	R	R	O
Haemochromatosis	O	O	O
Other liver diseases	R	Occ	O
Non-hepatic autoimmune diseases	VF	Occ	O
Drug-induced lupus/hepatitis	VF	F	F
Normal subjects (titres up to 1 : 80), (%)			
Age < 20 years	< 0·5	< 0·5	Very rare
20–40 years	< 3	< 1	but see
40–60 years	< 5	< 3	Table 6.2
> 60 years	≤ 25	< 5	

I, almost invariably (> 85%); VF, very frequently (60–85%); F, frequently (30–60%); Occ, occasionally (5–30%); R, rarely (1–5%); O, very rarely (< 1%); Var, reports vary widely; (T), transiently.
[a] With or without abnormal liver function tests.

the diagnostic criteria for AI-CAH. Certainly, this condition is associated with the highest frequency (60–85%) of ANA and SMA in liver disease (Table 6.5) and titres of 1 : 640 or greater are common. However, titres can fluctuate and the antibodies may even disappear without treatment.

Lower frequencies (15–40%) and generally lower titres of ANA and SMA are found in HBV-CAH and PBC than in AI-CAH (Table 6.5) and the antibodies are very rare in NANB-CAH [20]. In primary sclerosing cholangitis (PSC), the association with ANA and SMA is less clear. Most reports of routine screening by IF on tissue sections describe titres of ANA and SMA similar to those found in AI-CAH but with much lower frequency (<20%). However, a recent study [21] of autoantibodies in PSC sera, in which ANA were detected by IF not only on tissue sections but also using the HEp-2 cell line and *Crithidia luciliae* (Section 6.4.1), has found ANA and/or SMA at titres of 1 : 40 to 1 : 640 in up to 80% of the sera examined. The ANA were of the "homogeneous" type seen in SLE and AI-CAH. In contrast, ANA in PBC are often anti-centromere antibodies (Section 6.4.1), reflecting the frequent association of this disorder with one or more manifestations of the CREST syndrome. ANA of anti-Ro(SSA) or anti-La(SSB) specificity are also not uncommon in PBC due to its association with Sjogren's syndrome, in which these antibodies are prevalent (Section 6.4.1).

Mitochondrial antibodies (AMA) are considered to be characteristic of PBC and more than 95% of patients with this condition will be seropositive for AMA at some stage of their disease (Table 6.5). Titres of 1 : 2560 or greater are often seen. AMA occur infrequently in other disorders or in healthy subjects (even those of advanced age) and there is persuasive evidence to suggest that the majority of individuals who have no overt liver abnormality but are found to be seropositive for AMA at titres of 1 : 40 or greater may have underlying, asymptomatic PBC [19].

Approximately 20% of AMA-positive patients with chronic liver disease have clinical, biochemical and histological features that do not provide a clear distinction between AI-CAH and PBC. AMA in these overlap cases is of the M4 specificity (Section 6.4.3), which is distinct from the PBC-specific M2-AMA, but few laboratories routinely report on the sub-specificities of AMA at the present time. The clinical management of these overlap cases, with respect to whether or not to treat with corticosteroids, is a matter of continuing debate.

6.8.4   Liver autoantibodies

Apart from LKM (Section 6.4.4), the liver autoantibodies (i.e. those that are more specifically related to liver disease than are ANA or SMA, and the target antigens of which are largely of restricted organ distribution) do not usually form part of the autoantibody screen provided by most routine laboratories. However, testing for these autoantibodies can be very useful in diagnosis and for monitoring treatment.

The two liver–kidney microsomal antibodies (LKM-1 and LKM-2) are perhaps the best characterized. LKM-1 is found in a small but important sub-group of (usually young female) idiopathic CAH patients with particularly severe disease who are typically ANA and SMA seronegative. Unlike ANA and SMA, which usually reduce in titre and often disappear with response to corticosteroid treatment (sometimes never to reappear, even during relapses), titres of LKM-1

TABLE 6.6   Approximate frequencies of liver autoantibodies (see text) in various disorders

	LKM	Anti-LSP	Anti-ASGP-R	LMA	Anti-SLA	HMA
Chronic active hepatitis						
Autoimmune (untreated)	R	I	VF	VF	Occ	VF
HBV-related	O	VF	VF	Occ	O	VF
NANB-related	O	Occ	R	Var	O	F
Acute viral hepatitis						
Virus A or B	O	I (T)	F (T)	Occ	O	F
NANB viruses	O	Occ	O	Var	O	F
Other liver diseases						
Primary biliary cirrhosis	O	VF	Occ	F	O	I
Alcoholic liver disease	O	Occ	R	Occ	O	F
Primary sclerosing cholangitis	n.a.	Occ	R	n.a.	n.a.	n.a.
Wilson's disease	O	R	O	n.a.	n.a.	n.a.
Haemochromatosis	O	O	O	O	n.a.	n.a.
Drug-induced disorders	Occ	Occ	n.a.	F	O	I
Other	O	R	O	R	O	F
Non-hepatic autoimmune diseases	O	R	n.a.	R	O	R
Normal subjects	——		Very rarely and at low titres			——

n.a., Data not available; for other abbreviations and symbols see legend to Table 6.5.

tend to remain high. This might be related to the difficulty in controlling this severe form of idiopathic CAH with immunosuppressive drugs. LKM-2 antibodies are associated with drug-induced hepatitis and usually disappear when the condition resolves after withdrawal of the causative agent.

Anti-LSP, anti-ASGP-R and LMA (Sections 6.4.5 to 6.4.7) occur more frequently than LKM. Of the three, anti-LSP is perhaps the most extensively studied. It can be considered as a general marker of liver inflammation in certain disorders and its relative absence in others, such as NANB infections, Wilson's disease, haemochromatosis and toxic liver injury (Table 6.6), enhances its value as a diagnostic aid. In acute virus A (AVH-A) or B (AVH-B) hepatitis, almost all patients have high titres of anti-LSP during the early stages of their illnesses. Titres fall rapidly during recovery and patients usually become seronegative within three months. Failure of anti-LSP titres to fall appreciably within three months of an acute HBV infection is suggestive of progression to chronic liver disease.

In untreated CAH, titres of anti-LSP are proportional to the degree of periportal inflammation and piecemeal necrosis assessed histologically and are independent of serum biochemistry. Thus, anti-LSP is a useful guide to the severity of disease in the absence of a liver biopsy and can also be used to identify those HBV carriers with normal or only slightly abnormal LFTs who have underlying CAH (Chapter 5). Seropositivity for anti-LSP also identifies patients with PBC or alcoholic liver disease (ALD) who have histological features of CAH (periportal inflammation and piecemeal necrosis). The highest titres, however, are seen in AI-CAH. Titres decline and patients often become seronegative with response to corticosteroid therapy.

Patients who remain seropositive, and those in whom anti-LSP reappears, almost invariably relapse when corticosteroids are withdrawn. Rising titres can herald relapse five months or more before biochemical abnormalities appear [22]. These fluctuations in relation to the response to immunosuppressive therapy also make anti-LSP useful for monitoring compliance with treatment, which can be a particular problem in younger patients who are reluctant to take corticosteroids for long periods.

Anti-ASGP-R antibodies are more specific than anti-LSP for CAH but they do not discriminate between autoimmune (AI-) and HBV-related CAH. They occur much less frequently than anti-LSP in other liver diseases, such as PBC and ALD, and are extremely rare in NANB infections. Like anti-LSP, titres of anti-ASGP-R correlate well with histological activity in CAH, but they decline more rapidly with response to corticosteroids and reappear more slowly in advance of relapse when treatment is reduced or withdrawn. Thus, at the present time, it appears that anti-ASGP-R may be more specific than anti-LSP for the diagnosis of AI-CAH and HBV-CAH, but less useful for predicting relapse in patients on immunosuppressive treatment. Because of their frequency in AI-CAH and HBV-CAH and their rarity in NANB hepatitis and other disorders such as Wilson's disease, both anti-LSP and anti-ASGP-R may prove useful in the differential diagnosis of idiopathic CAH in patients who are seronegative for ANA and SMA.

LMA was originally thought to be a specific marker of AI-CAH but it is now known to occur with almost equal frequency in PBC as well as in ALD (Table 6.6). Its true value as a screening test is obscured by technical inconsistencies between studies in different laboratories, but most investigators agree that LMA is a marker of chronic liver disease (it seems to occur relatively infrequently in acute viral hepatitis, although this might be due to the difficulty of detecting LMA in sera that also contain immune complexes; see Section 6.4.5). Its usefulness as a prognostic index or for monitoring responses to treatment is uncertain owing to lack of serial studies to assess its value in this regard. Evidence relating to the occurrence of LMA in NANB infections is conflicting [10, 20], but it has been reported in up to 90% of patients with NANB-CAH and, if this is correct, it seems unlikely that this antibody could be used to discriminate between patients with chronic NANB infections and those with idiopathic CAH who are ANA/SMA-seronegative.

Two other liver autoantibodies, anti-SLA and HMA (Sections 6.4.8 and 6.4.9), have been described. Anti-SLA occurs in a small proportion of patients with idiopathic CAH, about 25% of whom are seronegative for ANA, SMA and LMA, but it is not known whether these patients are also negative for anti-LSP and/or anti-ASGP-R. Like anti-LSP and anti-ASGP-R, titres appear to fluctuate with response to corticosteroid treatment and anti-SLA may, therefore, prove useful for the monitoring of therapy in this small group of patients. In contrast, HMA is found in the majority of patients with AI-CAH, HBV-CAH or PBC. It also occurs frequently in AVH due to viruses A, B or NANB, as well as in a wide range of other liver disorders, including extrahepatic biliary obstruction, sarcoidosis, sclerosing cholangitis, haemochromatosis and Wilson's disease. In CAH, HMA is found more often in untreated patients than in those receiving corticosteroids, but it is not yet known whether this auto-antibody is of any value in monitoring therapy.

6.8.5 Other tests

Other seroimmunological parameters have generally proved to be of little practical clinical value to date in patients with liver disease. Circulating immune complexes (CIC), activation of complement and cryoglobulins in serum have all been widely reported in PBC but, although these abnormalities occur much less frequently in other liver disorders, they are not diagnostic of PBC. The latter disorder is a multisystem disease *par excellence*, with a strong association with the connective-tissue disorders and other conditions in which these serum abnormalities are common. Thus, it is likely that these serological features are related more to the associated (often asymptomatic) conditions in PBC than to the liver disease *per se*. On the other hand, since CIC will activate complement and can sometimes behave as cryoglobulins (which can cause many of the associated conditions such as vasculitis and Raynaud's phenomenon), it is possible that the CIC might be responsible for many of the extrahepatic manifestations of PBC. The origin and composition of the CIC in PBC is unknown, but there is evidence to suggest that they may be complexes of antigens derived from the biliary tract and their corresponding antibodies, which distinguishes them from CIC in SLE and rheumatoid arthritis [23]. CIC also occur in some patients with HBV-CAH and other hepatitis virus infections and, in these conditions, are thought to comprise viral antigens complexed to antiviral antibodies and may be associated with complement activation.

Notwithstanding the above, interest is reawakening in the measurement of circulating complement components and complement degradation products in patients with liver disease, particularly in relation to genetic disease associations in the immunopathological liver disorders, and some of these parameters may prove useful in clinical management when their value has been fully assessed.

As noted above (Section 6.7), acute phase reactants are too non-specific and variable to be a reliable aid in the diagnosis of liver disease, with the exception of those proteins (e.g. ferritin, prothrombin, ceruloplasmin) that are useful in other diagnostic contexts. However, techniques for measuring C-reactive protein (CRP) concentrations in plasma are now widely available and, as CRP levels fluctuate quite rapidly in relation to overall inflammatory activity, this acute-phase protein may be useful for monitoring early responses to therapy in patients with severe liver disease. In addition, measurements of serum amyloid-A component may be of value in amyloidosis involving the liver.

6.9 Technical notes

Immunology is still a relatively new discipline and several of the techniques that are applicable to clinical medicine are still evolving. At the present time, many of the seroimmunological parameters that are proving of value in diagnosis or monitoring of liver diseases are measured by different techniques in different laboratories. Since interpretation of a test result can often depend on precisely which method has been used, some knowledge of the methodological procedures is essential. The following technical notes have been written largely from the point of view of the detection of circulating antibodies (auto- or anti-microbial), but most of the techniques are also applicable to the detection of antigens in serum or in tissues by using specific antibodies raised in animals or produced by hybridoma technology.

6.9.1 Immunodiffusion and immunoelectrophoresis

Both immunodiffusion (ID) and immunoelectrophoresis (IEP) rely upon the diffusion, either passively (ID) or electrophoretically (IEP), of an antigen and antibody towards each other in a gel matrix (usually agar or agarose) to form a precipitin line at the point of equivalence. In the simplest systems, two wells punched in a 1–2-mm thick gel cast in a petri dish or on a glass slide are filled, one with a suitable dilution of the patient's serum and the other with a solution of the target antigen. After an appropriate period of incubation or electrophoresis, the gel is examined for precipitin lines and results are expressed usually only as positive or negative. A reasonable degree of quantitation can be achieved by performing the test with serial dilutions of the patient's serum or by using a modification of the basic technique whereby the gel is impregnated with the antigen and the patient's antibodies are allowed to migrate outwards from a single well cut in the gel. This is known as *radial ID*. The precipitin line forms a halo around the well containing the patient's serum and the area of the halo is directly proportional to the concentration of the antibody. ID and IEP are relatively easy and quick to perform but they are not very sensitive (no more so than IF, see below) and many autoantibodies do not give precipitin lines in these systems. Because of the low sensitivity and the need for a purified antigen for the test, ID and IEP are being used increasingly less often for the detection of autoantibodies.

6.9.1.1 Crossed immunoelectrophoresis
A variation on the above theme involves coupling simple electrophoresis with

IEP in a two-stage procedure. In the first step, the antigen is electrophoresed in a starch, agarose or polyacrylamide gel. The gel strip is then placed adjacent to a second gel which has been impregnated with the specific antiserum (or antibody-containing patient's serum) and electrophoresis is continued in a direction at right angles to the original direction. A two-dimensional picture of the resulting precipitin line(s) at the point of equivalence is thereby built up. The technique is particularly useful with impure antigen preparations or mixtures of antigens (e.g. for detecting specific serum proteins), but is rarely used for detecting autoantibodies.

6.9.2 Indirect immunofluorescence

Indirect immunofluorescence (IF) is the most commonly used technique for the routine detection of circulating autoantibodies. It is called *indirect* because a second antibody (an anti-immunoglobulin raised in animals) is used to detect the primary (patient's) antibody. An appropriate substrate (e.g. a tissue section) is incubated with a suitable dilution of the patient's serum, washed to remove non-adherent immunoglobulins and other serum proteins, then incubated with an anti-immunoglobulin which has been labelled with a fluorochrome (usually fluorescein or rhodamine) and after further washing is examined under ultraviolet light by using a fluorescence microscope. Most commonly, the substrate is a frozen section of rodent (mouse or rat) tissue that has been air-dried or has been fixed briefly with ethanol or acetone, but occasionally other fixatives or paraffin-embedded sections may be used. Alternatively, a tissue-culture cell line or a microbial culture may be employed.

The choice of substrate and fixative is very important, especially in the sub-classification of ANAs (see Section 6.4.1). Thus, a tissue-culture cell line (HEp-2 or KB cells) is required for detecting anti-centromere and anti-Ro(SSA) antibodies, Epstein–Barr virus-infected cells for antibodies against the rheumatoid arthritis-associated nuclear antigen (RANA), and *Crithidia luciliae* for anti-dsDNA, while the Ro(SSA) antigen is easily solubilized (even by ethanol or methanol) and antibodies reacting with it may be missed by inappropriate treatment of the substrate. The advantages of IF are its relative ease and rapidity of performance and its lack of requirement for a purified antigen. The main disadvantages relate to the wide intra- and inter-laboratory variations in the substrates and the need for an experienced observer for interpretation, which is largely subjective and liable to inter-observer variation.

6.9.2.1 Avidin–biotin based systems

Avidin is a glycoprotein derived from the whites of avian eggs that has a high affinity for the vitamin biotin. Both avidin and biotin can be fairly easily coupled covalently to many proteins and other molecules. These two properties have been widely exploited to modify and increase the sensitivities of many immunoassays. Thus, in immunofluorescence systems, the anti-immunoglobulin is coupled to biotin and the fluorochrome is linked to avidin. After incubation of the patient's serum with the substrate, the biotinylated anti-immunoglobulin is added followed by the avidin-fluorochrome. Since many biotin molecules can be coupled to each anti-immunoglobulin molecule, many avidin-fluorochrome molecules can bind to each anti-immunoglobulin, thereby considerably enhancing the fluorescence when the substrate is viewed under ultraviolet light. There are numerous variations on this basic principle. For example, the avidin can be coupled to an enzyme (alkaline phosphatase, peroxidase) that produces a colour reaction with an appropriate chemical substrate and the resulting colour reaction can be examined by normal light microscopy. Avidin-linked enzymes have also been used in ELISA systems (see below).

6.9.2.2 Quantitative immunofluorescence

Quantitative immunofluorescence has more in common with ELISAs (see below) than with the method of indirect immunofluorescence described above. When used for detection of serum autoantibodies, it depends on the availability of a purified target antigen (e.g. DNA) which can be attached to a solid phase (e.g. a plastic bead). Appropriate dilutions of the test serum are incubated with the immobilized antigen and autoantibodies binding to it are detected by using a fluorochrome-labelled anti-immunoglobulin. The fluorescence is measured in a specially designed microfluorimeter and is directly proportional to the amount of autoantibody that has bound to the solid phase antigen. The advantages of the system are essentially the same as those of ELISAs. The main disadvantages relate to the cost of the equipment and the limitations imposed by the need for a purified antigen.

6.9.3 Enzyme-linked immunosorbent assays

The basic principle of enzyme-linked immunosorbent assays (ELISAs) for autoantibodies is similar to that of IF except that the target antigen is usually (and preferably) highly purified and the second antibody (the anti-immunoglobulin) is linked to an enzyme (usually alkaline phosphatase or peroxidase) which is capable of catalysing a colour reaction with an appropriate chemical substrate (the chromogen). In almost all simple ELISA systems, the target antigen is immobilized by attaching it to a plastic surface (the solid phase) such as a plastic bead or the well of a microtitre plate. Attachment is achieved by electrostatic or covalent bonding but, increasingly, more complex systems are being devised in which, for example, an antibody (often monoclonal) raised in animals against the specific antigen is attached to the plastic surface and this is then used to immobilize the antigen. To perform the test, an appropriate dilution of the patient's serum is added and after a suitable incubation period (followed by extensive washing) adherent antibodies are detected by adding the enzyme-linked anti-immunoglobulin followed by the chromogen. The intensity of colour which develops by interaction of the enzyme with its substrate can be determined visually (by comparison with appropriate standards) or, more precisely by spectrophotometry, and is directly proportional to the amount of specific autoantibody in the patient's serum. The results are expressed using a scoring system (when visual assessment is employed) or, when determined spectrophotometrically, as arbitrary antibody units or as titres (related to the dilution of the patient's serum that was used).

The advantages of ELISAs are their sensitivity (10^2 to 10^3 times more sensitive than IF), objectivity (when results are determined spectrophotometrically) and facility for semi-automation. However, when used for the detection of autoantibodies in disease, they are prone to artefacts and quite complicated safeguards are required to avoid false-positive results.

6.9.4 Dot-immunobinding assays

Dot-immunobinding assays are a variation of the ELISA principle. A drop of a solution containing the purified target antigen is placed on a nitrocellulose sheet and dried to allow the antigen to become attached to the nitrocellulose. A drop of the patient's serum (appropriately diluted) is then placed on top of the antigen "dot" and, after a suitable incubation period, the sheet is washed thoroughly. Antibodies binding to the antigen "dot" are detected by adding an enzyme-linked anti-immunoglobulin followed by the appropriate chromogen (as for ELISAs) and reading the resulting colour reaction visually. A reasonable approximation of the amount of antibody can be made by using serial dilutions of the patient's serum and suitable standards. The method has the advantages of rapidity and relative simplicity, but it is at best only semiquantitative and great care is required to avoid false-positive results due to non-specific binding of immunoglobulins to the nitrocellulose. So far, this technique has been shown to be useful only for a small number of antibodies that occur at relatively high titres in serum.

6.9.5 Radioimmunoassays

Radioimmunoassays (RIA) is a generic term covering a wide range of techniques in which at least one component of the system is labelled with a radioactive isotope. When used for detection of autoantibodies, the basic principle involves either the detection of immune complexes formed by interacting the patient's antibody-containing serum with a purified radio-labelled target antigen or the determination of the degree of inhibition (by the patient's antibody) of the binding of a radiolabelled antibody (e.g. raised in animals) to an appropriate unlabelled antigen. Alternatively, the assay may employ a solid-phase system similar to that of ELISAs (see above) in which patients' autoantibodies that bind to the immobilized target antigen are detected by a radiolabelled anti-immunoglobulin.

One of the earliest RIAs to be adopted for routine use was the Farr assay. This depends on the fact that many antigens are soluble in 50% saturated ammonium sulphate solution but immunoglobulins tend not to be. Thus, after incubation of radiolabelled antigen with the patient's serum, addition of 50% saturated anmonium sulphate allows separation of free antigen (which remains in solution) from antigen–antibody complexes which assume the solubility characteristics of the antibody and are precipitated. However, the technical variations on this and other RIAs, such as the radioallergosorbent test (RAST) for detection of specific IgE antibodies, are too numerous to be covered adequately here and the reader is referred to specialized texts (see Section 6.11) for further information. RIAs have the advantage of very high sensitivity, which is comparable to (or often greater than) that of ELISAs and, like ELISAs, can be semi-automated. Disadvantages include the requirement for expensive counting equipment and the relatively short shelf-life (2–12 weeks) of the radiolabelled components in many RIA systems. In addition, because the systems are so highly sensitive, rigorous standardization is essential.

6.9.6 Haemagglutination assays

A wide variety of assays based on the ability of antibodies to agglutinate mammalian or avian erythrocytes that have been coated with corresponding antigens is available. Coating can be achieved by spontaneous coupling when the red cells are added to a solution of the antigen but usually "sensitization" of the cells by brief exposure to formalin, tannic acid, glutaraldehyde or other agents (e.g. chromium chloride, carbodiimide) is required as a preliminary step to coupling with the antigen. The assay is customarily performed in an 80- or 96-well microtitre plate. To each row of wells is added serial dilutions of a serum under test, followed by the suspension of coated red cells, with the final well in each row being reserved for testing the serum at the lowest dilution against uncoated red cells (to exclude false-positive results due to non-specific agglutinins in the patient's serum). The testing of serial dilutions is important because sera with high titres of specific autoantibodies (particularly those of IgM class) tend to exhibit a prozone effect, i.e. giving a negative result at low dilutions. The end-point is taken as the highest dilution at which definite agglutination of the red cells is observed and the result is expressed in terms of this dilution point as a titre.

The technique described above is termed "passive" or "indirect" haemagglutination to distinguish it from assays for agglutinating antibodies that react directly with red cell antigens (e.g. agglutination of group-A erythrocytes by anti-A sera). For non-agglutinating autoantibodies, the test can be modified by using a second antibody (an anti-immunoglobulin raised in an animal) to achieve agglutination. In that event, the assay is performed as a two-stage procedure in which the antigen-coated cells are incubated first with serial dilutions of the patient's serum then with the anti-immunoglobulin. The sensitivity of these assays is intermediate between that of ID, IEP or IF and that of ELISAs or RIAs. Additional advantages include their relative ease and rapidity of performance and the reasonably quantitative results obtained. Sensitivity and precision can be increased by coupling the test to a complement-fixing haemolytic assay (see below) but, since the haemagglutination assays require purified antigens for specific detection of auto-antibodies, they have largely been replaced by the more objective and highly sensitive ELISA or RIA systems when such antigen preparations are available.

6.9.7 Complement-fixation tests

Complement-fixation tests are two-stage tests in which the first step is essentially the same as for a haemagglutination assay, except that the tests are usually performed in tubes rather than microtitre plates. After incubation with the patient's serum, the antigen-coated erythrocytes are washed and guinea-pig complement is added. The haemoglobin released during the consequent complement-mediated lysis of those red cells to which the patient's autoantibodies have become attached is determined spectrophotometrically and is directly proportional to the number of cells lysed and, if the system has been properly standardized, can be related fairly precisely to the amount of autoantibody that was bound. Results may be expressed as arbitrary antibody units or as titres related to the highest dilution of the patient's serum that gives a predefined amount of haemoglobin release in the assay. Several very sensitive assays have been developed on this principle by miniaturizing the system and by using highly purified antigens. As a general rule, however, they tend to be a little too cumbersome for routine autoantibody screening.

6.9.8 Nephelometry

Nephelometry is the measurement of the light scattered when a beam is passed through a solution. The term must be distinguished from turbidimetry, which measures the decrease in light passing through a cloudy solution. When antigens and antibodies combine, the resulting immune complexes can cause light passing through the solution to be deflected and this is the basis for the use of nephelometry in immunoassays. The principle has been in use for many years but recent advances in the electronic detection of the scattered light and other improvements have greatly enhanced its accuracy and sensitivity. In addition, the technique lends itself to automation and for this reason is widely employed for the measurement of serum immunoglobulins and other serum proteins which can be detected by using specific antisera. Disadvantages include the cost of the equipment and the fact that, as accurate measurements can only be made in antigen excess, multiple dilutions of the sample may need to be tested. However, modern equipment overcomes this latter problem by testing serial dilutions automatically.

References

1. Gurian LE *et al*. Hepatology 1985; 5: 397.
2. Lidman K. Acta Med Scand 1976; 200: 403.
3. Andersen P. Acta Pathol Microbiol Scand, Sect C 1979; 87: 110.
4. Rizetto M *et al*. Clin Exp Immunol 1973; 15: 331.
5. Odievre M *et al*. Hepatology 1983; 3: 407.
6. Alvarez F *et al*. J Exp Med 1985; 161: 1231.
7. Beaune P *et al*. Proc Nat Acad Sci USA 1987; 84: 551.
8. Hopf U *et al*. N Engl J Med 1976; 294: 578.
9. Gerken G *et al*. J Hepatol 1987; 5: 65.
10. McFarlane IG and Williams R. J Hepatol 1985; 1: 313.
11. McFarlane IG. Clin Sci 1983; 64: 127.

12. McFarlane IG *et al.* Clin Exp Immunol 1984; 55: 347.
13. Manns M *et al.* Lancet 1987; i: 292.
14. Lee WM *et al.* Clin Exp Immunol 1985; 62: 715.
15. Lawley TJ *et al.* Gastroenterology 1980; 78: 626.
16. Abrass CK *et al.* Clin Exp Immunol 1980; 40: 292.
17. Wands JR *et al.* Gastroenterology 1975; 69: 1286.
18. Potter BJ *et al.* J Lab Clin Med 1976; 88: 427.
19. Mitchison HC *et al.* Hepatology 1986; 6: 1279.
20. Mackay IR *et al.* Clin Exp Immunol 1985; 61: 39.
21. Zauli D *et al.* J Hepatol 1987; 5: 14.
22. McFarlane IG *et al.* Lancet 1984; ii: 954.
23. Amoroso P *et al.* Clin Exp Immunol 1980; 42: 95.

Suggested further reading

Andersen P. Incidence and titres of smooth muscle antibodies in human sera. Acta Pathol Microbiol Scand, Sect C 1979; 87: 11–16.

Baltz ML and Pepys MB. Acute phase proteins with special reference to C-reactive protein and related proteins (pentaxins) and serum amyloid A protein. Adv Immunol 1983; 34: 141–212.

Baum H and Palmer C. The PBC-specific antigen. In: Molecular Aspects of Primary Biliary Cirrhosis (Epstein O, Ed). Mol Asp Med 1985; 8: 201–234.

Berg PA and Klein R. Clinical and prognostic relevance of different mitochondrial antibody profiles in primary biliary cirrhosis (PBC). In: Molecular Aspects of Primary Biliary Cirrhosis (Epstein O, Ed). Mol Asp Med 1985; 8: 235–247.

Endo L, Corman LCC and Panush RS. Clinical utility of assays for circulating immune complexes. Med Clin North Am 1985; 69: 623–636.

Harmon CE. Antinuclear antibodies in autoimmune disease. Med Clin North Am 1985; 69: 547–563.

Homberg JC, Abuaf N, Bernard O *et al.* Chronic active hepatitis associated with anti-liver/kidney microsome antibody type 1: A second type of "autoimmune" hepatitis. Hepatology 1987; 7: 1333–1339.

Langone JJ and Van Vunakis H. Immunochemical techniques, Part B. Methods in Enzymology Vol. 73 (Colowick SP and Kaplan NO, Eds). New York: Academic Press, 1981.

Lidman K. Clinical diagnosis in patients with smooth muscle antibodies. Acta Med Scand 1976; 200: 403–407.

McFarlane IG. Autoimmunity in liver disease. Clin Sci 1984; 67: 569–578.

McFarlane IG and Williams R. Liver membrane antibodies. J Hepatol 1985; 1: 313–319.

Reeves G. Lecture Notes on Immunology. Oxford: Blackwell, 1987.

Stites DP, Stobo JD and Wells JV. (Eds). Basic and Clinical Immunology, 6th edn. Los Altos, California: Appleton & Lange, 1987.

Tan EM. Autoantibodies to nuclear antigens (ANA). Adv Immunol 1982; 33: 167–240.

Van Vunakis H and Langone JJ. Immunochemical techniques, Part A. Methods in Enzymology, Vol. 70 (Colowick SP and Kaplan NO, Eds). New York: Academic Press, 1980.

Weir DM. (Ed). Handbook of Experimental Immunology, Vols 1–3 3rd edn. Oxford: Blackwell, 1978.

7

Endocrine abnormalities

7.1   Introduction

In this chapter we are concerned with four aspects of the interface between liver disease and endocrinology. Firstly, chronic liver disease can lead to endocrine dysfunction in its own right, although the role of alcohol which can cause both chronic liver disease and endocrine disturbances complicates matters. Secondly, some primary endocrine diseases can affect liver function. Thirdly, diseases such as haemo-chromatosis (Chapter 11) involve both the liver and the endocrine system, and, finally, endocrine and liver diseases may co-exist as a result of sharing common mechanisms of pathogenesis. The major challenge to the clinician is the correct application and interpretation of the standard endocrine investigations in patients with liver disease.

7.2 Sex hormones and their binding proteins [1]

Men with cirrhosis are frequently impotent, infertile and feminized (i.e. they may have gynaecomastia, a female distribution of body hair and testicular atrophy). Workers in the United States, where alcohol is responsible for a very high percentage of all chronic liver disease, have tended to attribute these symptoms to the alcohol rather than the chronic liver disease. In the UK where at least 50% of patients with cirrhosis have non-alcohol related disease, sexual dysfunction is still seen and it seems most likely that alcohol may act both on its own, and in concert with chronic liver disease, to cause sexual dysfunction. The biochemical and endocrine changes which accompany chronic liver disease are now well recognized but they correlate poorly with the clinical symptoms. The section describes the changes in endocrine tests which might be expected in patients with liver disease of various aetiologies and severity, but it is important to note that the changes described are not necessarily the cause of symptoms. The discussion below refers mainly to men; the effect of liver disease on sexual function in women has been less studied.

7.2.1 Physiology and biochemistry

The major circulating androgen is testosterone secreted by the testicular Leydig cells ($5-10$ mg day^{-1} under the control of interstitial-cell stimulating hormone [identical to, and more often referred to as, luteinizing hormone (LH)]. The androgenic effect of androstenedione and other adrenal androgens such as dehydroepiandrosterone is probably attributable to their peripheral conversion to testosterone. Testosterone may be metabolized to its

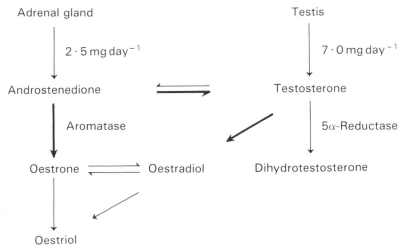

FIG. 7.1 Pathways for the production of oestrogens and androgens in males. The bold lines represent those pathways which are enhanced in patients with cirrhosis.

more active metabolite dihydrotestosterone (DHT, by 5α reduction), or to oestrogens (by the enzyme aromatase), or by degradation in the liver which is responsible for clearing about 50% of testosterone during the first pass in males. Oestrogens also circulate in men, the most potent being oestradiol (strictly, 17β-oestradiol, but more often referred to as E2) which is derived from aromatization of testosterone (Fig 7.1). Testosterone and oestradiol circulate bound to albumin (low affinity, unsaturable binding) and sex-hormone binding globulin (SHBG, high affinity, saturable binding). Only a small amount exists in the unbound state and this is presumed to be the biologically active fraction.

Spermatogenesis proceeds under the control of follicle stimulating hormone (FSH) although LH is also required, acting indirectly on the seminiferous tubules by stimulating testosterone secretion by the adjacent Leydig cells.

7.2.2. Changes in men with cirrhosis [1,2]

The total serum testosterone concentration is at the lower limit of the reference range in most men with well-compensated liver disease and falls as the disease progresses. The oestradiol concentration, on the other hand, is usually at the upper limit of the reference range and *rises* as the disease progresses and the ratio of oestradiol : testosterone is thus elevated. Because SHBG levels are invariably also raised, and the affinity with which testosterone is bound is considerably greater than that of oestradiol. The ratio of free-oestrogen : testosterone is even greater.

The low testosterone levels are attributable to reduced testicular production and occur despite a decrease in metabolic clearance rate caused by the high SHBG levels. The elevated oestrogen levels are not due to impaired hepatic clearance as originally thought; increased production, probably due to enhanced peripheral aromatization, appears to be the most likely mechanism.

In the presence of low testosterone levels, a compensatory increase in pituitary secretion of LH would be expected, but this does not always occur, implying that a primary testicular defect is often complicated by hypothalamic–pituitary dysfunction. As the disease progresses, LH levels tend to fall. Thus the characteristic abnormalities may be represented as a spectrum (Table 7.1). Similar but less pronounced changes also occur in post-menopausal women with chronic liver disease [3].

Three-quarters of men with cirrhosis have oligospermia and this is associated with normal levels of FSH. Absence of testicular atrophy, a normal LH, or a normal LH or FSH response to clomiphene or gonadotrophin-releasing hormone (GnRH) predict recovery of sexual function in alcoholic men who abstain from further drinking [4].

Hypogonadism is a prominent feature in men with idiopathic haemochromatosis (Chapter 11) [5]. Unlike the situation with other types of cirrhosis, such as that due to alcohol, impotence may occur very early in the disease (even before the cirrhosis develops). It is probably due to a combination of testicular damage due to iron overload (and excessive alcohol consumption, often a feature of haemochromatosis), pituitary dysfunction,

TABLE 7.1   Changes in the plasma sex hormone concentrations in men with chronic liver disease in relation to its severity (Chapter 1)

	Well compensated cirrhosis	Poorly compensated cirrhosis
Testosterone (T)	Low/normal	Low
Oestradiol (E_2)	High/normal	High
SHBG	High	High
Total E_2/T	High	Very high
LH	Normal	Low

LH, leutinizing hormone; SHBG, sex-hormone binding globulin.

concurrent hepatic cirrhosis and diabetic autonomic neuropathy. The pituitary dysfunction, which is probably the most important factor, is caused by selective iron deposition in the gonadotrophin-secreting cells. Levels of LH (and prolactin) are subnormal in the majority of men with clinical hypogonadism.

7.2.3 Changes in liver function during pregnancy [6]

Abnormalities (occasionally marked) in the liver function tests may occur during normal pregnancy. These have been attributed, not unreasonably, to changes in the hormonal environment, and there is good experimental evidence that oestrogens are involved. Thus similar abnormalities are also seen in women taking the contraceptive pill or challenged with oestrogenic preparations.

The most pronounced change is a tendency towards cholestasis (Chapters 1 and 2) in the last trimester. Normally this can only be detected by very sensitive techniques such as the bromsulphthalein (BSP) excretion test (Chapter 3), but lipid concentrations also increase. The serum activities of GGTP and alkaline phosphatase also rise in late pregnancy but the latter is attributable mainly to *placental* alkaline phosphatase (Chapter 2). In a small percentage of women, however, this tendency is exaggerated and symptoms of jaundice and/or pruritus develop. Although different names are given depending on the predominant symptom, they probably form part of a spectrum (Table 7.2). Signs and symptoms disappear within a few

TABLE 7.2 Laboratory investigations in normal pregnant women and in those with intrahepatic cholestasis of pregnancy

	Serum bilirubin	AST[a]	ALP	BSP retention	Pruritus
Normal pregnancy	Normal	Normal	High	Increased	No
Pruritus gravidarum	Normal	$1-2 \times N$	High	Increased	Yes
Recurrent jaundice of pregnancy	Increased	$2-4 \times N$	High	Increased	Yes

[a] N, upper limit of reference range.
AST, aspartate aminotransferase; ALP, alkaline phosphatase.

days, or even hours, of delivery but recur with varying degrees of severity in subsequent pregnancies or on exposure to oestrogen either therapeutically or in contraceptive preparations. Female relatives of patients with *intrahepatic cholestasis of pregnancy* (as the whole syndrome is now often classified) are at an increased risk of developing the same syndrome.

Acute fatty liver of pregnancy is another condition specific to pregnancy but may be much more severe. The patient usually becomes jaundiced, AST levels are markedly elevated and hepatic failure often ensues. Patients with preeclampsia may develop liver damage and very high levels of AST, although in this condition serum bilirubin levels are usually normal.

Not surprisingly, the excretory defect in patients with the Dubin–Johnson syndrome (see 2.5.2 and 11.9.2) is worsened by oestrogens and such patients often first present with, or suffer from, increasing jaundice during pregnancy or on first exposure to the contraceptive pill. Pregnancy and the contraceptive pill are also associated with the development of benign liver tumours and increased blood coagulability leading to hepatic-vein thrombosis (Chapter 4), but both of these complications are exceedingly rare.

7.3 Thyroid hormones and their binding proteins

Patients with chronic liver disease, particularly alcoholic cirrhosis, often have prominent, staring eyes which at first sight appear exophthalmic and the simple serum tests of thyroid function, serum triiodothyronine (T_3), thyroxine (T_4), and thyroid stimulating hormone (TSH) are frequently abnormal. This can give the impression of thyrotoxicosis. Nonetheless, on more-detailed examination and investigation by the appropriate tests (Section 7.3.3) the great majority will be found to be euthyroid. It is therefore important to recognize that conventional tests of thyroid function must be interpreted with considerable caution in the presence of chronic liver disease.

7.3.1 Physiology and biochemistry

The thyroid gland, under the influence of TSH, secretes about 100 nmol day^{-1} of T_4 and 5 nmol day^{-1} of T_3. TSH is itself controlled by thyrotrophin-releasing factor (TRH) from the hypothalamus, and both are part of a

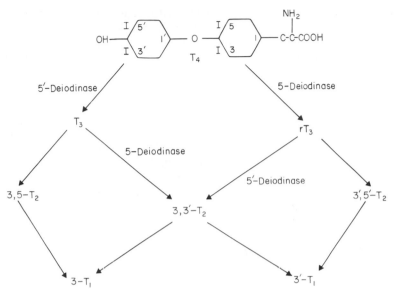

FIG. 7.2   Catabolism of thyroxine. 5'-Deiodinase is an hepatic enzyme and hence in liver disease T_3 levels are low and rT_3 levels raised.

feedback system completed by the thyroid hormones. In the liver, thyroxine may be deiodinated, conjugated and secreted in the bile, or deaminated. Deiodination is the major pathway and proceeds as a series of monodeiodination steps involving two enzymes (5-deiodinase and 5'-deiodinase). 5'-Deiodination results in the formation of the more metabolically active T_3; conversion of T_4 to the metabolically inactive reverse T_3 (rT_3) (5-deiodination) occurs at extrahepatic sites (Fig. 7.2). Thyroid hormones circulate bound to three proteins — throxine-binding globulin (TBG), prealbumin and albumin — all of which are synthesized by the liver, and as with the sex hormones, only the small unbound fractions of the thyroid hormones are considered to be metabolically active.

7.3.2   Changes in acute liver disease

Thyroid function in acute hepatitis has been studied [7] but the results are largely of academic interest as it is very unlikely that a diagnosis of hyperthyroidism during acute hepatitis would ever be entertained. Nonetheless, serum thyroxine levels are often increased and this has been attributed to high TBG levels, as a result of release of the protein from damaged hepatocytes. Patients with acute hepatitis have no clinical signs of hyperthyroidism (other than loss of weight) and free thyroxine and serum TSH (measured using a sensitive immuno-radiometric assay) will be within the reference range as will the TSH response to TRH.

7.3.3   Changes in chronic liver disease

In chronic liver disease the rate of thyroxine secretion and its serum level are usually normal. Where abnormal values (whether high or low) occur, they are often attributable to abnormalities of serum concentration of TBG (Fig. 7.3). Elevated levels of TBG occur in about 40% of patients with cirrhosis in whom this is complicated by hepatocellular carcinoma (Chapter 8) and in about 5–10% of those with uncomplicated cirrhosis, particularly primary biliary cirrhosis and chronic active hepatitis [8]. This may lead to very high levels of serum T_4 despite the patient being clinically euthyroid. On the other hand, as cirrhosis becomes decompensated and the synthetic capacity of the liver falls, T_3 and T_4 levels may fall in parallel with TBG.

There is depression of 5'-iodinase activity in cirrhosis which results in a decrease of T_4 to T_3 conversion and also a decrease in rT_3 deiodination (See

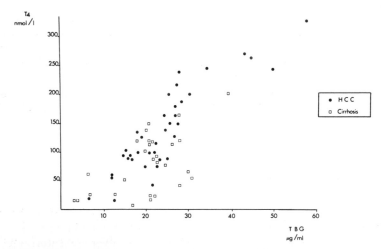

FIG. 7.3   Relationship of thyroxine to thyroxine binding globulin in patients with cirrhosis or hepatocellular carcinoma.

Fig 7.2) leading to a low T_3/rT_3 ratio which is characteristic of decompensated liver disease, but also of several other chronic, non-thyroidal illnesses [9].

7.3.4 Primary thyroidal illness in chronic liver disease

As a rule, high or low serum levels of T_3 and T_4 in patients with chronic liver disease simply reflect abnormal values of serum TBG and most will be euthyroid. The situation may, however, be complicated by true thyroid dysfunction (there is a high incidence of hyper- and hypothyroidism amongst patients with chronic active hepatitis or primary biliary cirrhosis [10]). In these situations, direct estimation of free thyroxine, serum TSH (measured by immunoradiometric assay) or an index which takes into account TBG levels (such as the T_4/TBG ratio) will usually give the appropriate result [11]. Both basal and stimulated TSH levels are normal in cirrhosis without thyroid dysfunction as are other, physiological indices of thyroid function such as the Achilles reflex time.

7.3.5 Abnormalities of liver function in primary thyroid disease

Patients with thyrotoxicosis may occasionally have slight and non-specific abnormalities of liver function tests (LFTs), usually a raised alkaline phosphatase activity (of liver origin). Jaundice has been described but this is usually due to associated cardiac failure (Chapter 2) or secondary to thyroid crisis, a syndrome which is seldom encountered nowadays. Thyrotoxicosis may also precipitate jaundice in patients with Gilbert's syndrome and jaundice is a feature of neonatal hypothyroidism (Chapter 2).

7.3.6 Prognostic implications

In common with many chronic diseases, as the cirrhotic process progresses, levels of T_3 fall and levels of rT_3 rise. A high rT_3/T_3 ratio is a particularly bad prognostic sign in chronic liver disease and indicates a survival of less than three months in more than 75% of such patients [9].

7.4 Glucose metabolism

Patients with chronic liver disease frequently exhibit glucose intolerance, and this may be detected even before the liver disease is recognized. In patients with severe acute liver disease hypoglycaemia may be life threatening. In the light of the central role of the liver in glucose and insulin metabolism, reviewed briefly below, disturbances of carbohydrate homeostasis in liver disease are not surprising.

7.4.1 Physiology and biochemistry

The liver acts as a reservoir for glucose. At times of plenty, during and immediately after feeding, it stores glucose as glycogen (which may be converted to triglycerides) and then releases glucose as required during the period between meals. Insulin, which is secreted directly into the portal–venous system, is the major stimulus to such storage. This hormone lowers blood sugar by reducing hepatic glycogenolysis and gluconeogenesis as well as stimulating peripheral uptake and utilization. These actions are opposed by counter-regulatory hormones including glucagon (which stimulates hepatic glucose production), growth hormone, cortisol, and catecholamines.

7.4.2 Glucose intolerance in chronic liver disease [12]

Most patients with cirrhosis exhibit a characteristic triad of abnormalities when challenged with a glucose load, either orally or intravenously (Fig. 7.4), namely hyperglycaemia, hyperinsulinaemia and hyperglucagonaemia. Under fasting conditions hyperglycaemia is much less common (less than 5%) although the high insulin levels may still be detectable and hyperglucagonaemia is also a consistent feature. The high hormone levels are caused by pancreatic hypersecretion but may be increased still further, particularly after a glucose load, by reduced hepatic extraction and portal-systemic shunting [13].

Glucose intolerance seldom causes any symptoms and does not usually require treatment. Indeed it has been suggested that when fasting hyperglycaemia occurs "true", i.e. idiopathic, diabetes mellitus is co-existent with liver disease and this is considered to be the case in the small minority of patients with liver disease who require insulin. The situation may not be, however, so clear-cut. Most

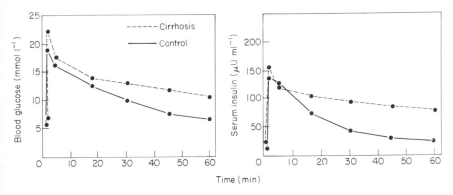

FIG. 7.4   Typical intravenous glucose tolerance test in a patient with cirrhosis (----) compared to a normal subject (————).

cirrhotics who require insulin develop this requirement late in adult life after gradually decreasing glucose tolerance rather than presenting acutely with ketoacidosis and do not seem to develop the complication of classical diabetes mellitus.

On the other hand, patients with haemochromatosis do develop typical diabetes mellitus (Chapter 11) [14]. In addition to the mechanisms described above, and more importantly, these patients have impaired insulin secretion due to pancreatic disease and develop similar complications to classical insulin dependent diabetes mellitus.

Glucose intolerance in patients with chronic liver disease is frequently exacerbated by treatment with corticosteroids. Whilst hypoglycaemia is the characteristic feature of fulminant hepatic failure, about 10% of patients develop hyperglycaemia during the course of the illness for reasons which are not clear.

7.4.3   Liver function in idiopathic diabetes mellitus

Liver function tests (LFTs) are normal in well-controlled diabetes; in poorly controlled patients a mildly elevated alkaline phosphatase activity is common, perhaps reflecting hepatic steatosis. Oral hypoglycaemic agents may cause cholestatic jaundice, the most commonly implicated being chlorpropamide (Chapter 9). Other reasons which cause diabetic patients to develop abnormalities of liver function include gallstones and cirrhosis (both of which are increased in frequency in idiopathic diabetes mellitus).

7.4.4 Hypoglycaemia in liver disease

Hypoglycaemia is a frequent and a potentially lethal complication of fulminant hepatitis and in children with Reye's syndrome and glycogen storage diseases. Other hepatic conditions in which episodic hypoglycaemia may occur include hereditary fructose intolerance and galactosaemia (Chapter 11). Given the importance of the liver in glucose homeostasis under normal circumstances (it is the sole source of endogenous glucose production), hypoglycaemia is remarkably uncommon in patients with chronic liver disease but may occur occasionally in patients with alcoholic cirrhosis after a binge and is attributable to inhibition of gluconeogenesis. Hypoglycaemia is an occasional complication of hepatocellular carcinoma and of large and rapidly growing secondary liver tumours (Chapter 8).

7.5 Vitamin D and calcium metabolism

Disturbances of calcium and phosphate metabolism are infrequent in chronic liver disease, although calcium levels tend to be low because of co-existent hypoalbuminaemia (see Chapter 2) and high in patients with some hepatic malignancies (Chapter 8). On the other hand, bone disease is recognized to be a major problem. This usually takes the form of *osteoporosis*, in which there is a reduction in bone mass. The aetiology is not known, but it is recognized to be exacerbated by corticosteroid administration which is widely used in some forms of liver disease, such as chronic active hepatitis and following liver transplantation.

Recently, however, as the mechanisms of action of vitamin D have become better understood, the extent of *osteomalacia* (abnormal mineralization of bone) in chronic liver disease has been examined in more detail because the liver is the site of the initial activation step of vitamin D (Fig 7.5).

It seemed likely, therefore, that patients with liver disease might not be able to hydroxylate vitamin D_3 and that osteomalacia might result. Indeed it was widely reported that up to 75% of patients with cholestatic liver disease such as primary biliary cirrhosis or sclerosing cholangitis had evidence of osteomalacia [15]. However, when the most rigid diagnostic criteria were applied (increased mean osteoid width measured directly, together with an increase in the mineraliz-

Hydroxylation   Hydroxylation

$$\text{Vitamin D}_3 \dashrightarrow 25\text{-(OH)}_2\text{D}_3 \dashrightarrow 1, 25\text{-(OH)}_2\text{D}_3$$

(Liver)   (Kidney)   The active metabolite

FIG. 7.5 Activation pathway of vitamin D_3.

ation lag time — the time interval between apposition and subsequent mineralization of osteoid as derived from tetracycline labelling), no evidence of osteomalacia was found [16]. Thus, in all but the most severe degrees of cholestatic liver disease, the hydroxylation of vitamin D_3 proceeds normally and levels of 25-(OH)$_2$D$_3$ are normal. Osteoporosis and not osteomalacia is the major form of bone pathology in patients with liver disease [16]. If vitamin D treatment is indicated it is important to monitor fasting uncuffed plasma calcium and phosphate and 25-(OH)D, the concentration of which should be maintained in the upper part of the reference range.

7.6 Adrenal function

There are no consistent, clinically significant, disturbances of adrenal function in chronic liver disease. However, cortisol-binding globulin levels may be low. This is said to lead to higher free concentrations of prednisolone in patients treated with corticosteroids, and may be responsible for the observation that patients with liver disease seem to develop Cushingoid features at relatively low doses of corticosteroid drugs.

A situation in which diagnostic confusion often arises is *pseudo-Cushing's syndrome* which may be seen in patients with alcoholic cirrhosis [17]. Alcohol consumption rather than liver disease is probably the most important aetiological factor. The patient presents with the clinical appearance of Cushing's syndrome: muscle wasting, easy bruising, "buffalo hump", glucose intolerance and a moon face (which may be accentuated by the parotid enlargement often seen in cirrhotics). Plasma cortisol and ACTH levels are elevated, both lose their normal diurnal rhythm and cortisol levels are not suppressed by dexamethasone. There are thus clinical and biochemical features which are entirely compatible with a diagnosis of Cushing's syndrome. The syndrome is presumed to be due to chronic adrenal stimulation by alcohol complicated by the fact that many of the clinical signs of

Cushing's syndrome and cirrhosis are similar. However, after a few days abstinence from alcohol, all biochemical the abnormalities disappear, and hence the term *pseudo* Cushing's syndrome.

7.6.1 Aldosterone

Although representing only a tiny fraction of the total adrenal steroid production, aldosterone may be of considerable importance in the pathogenesis of ascites (Chapter 3). The high concentrations of aldosterone characteristic of cirrhotics who are retaining sodium is caused by activation of the renin–angiotensin system. Measurement of these hormones is not of any diagnostic value.

References

1. Johnson PJ. Clin Sci 1984; 66: 369.
2. Bannister P and Losowsky MS. J Hepatol 1988; 6: 258.
3. Bannister P, *et al*. Clin Endocrinol 1985; 23: 335.
4. Van Thiel DH, *et al*. Gastroenterology 1982; 84: 677.
5. Walton C, *et al*. Quart J Med, New Ser LII 1983; 205: 99.
6. Van Thiel DH (Ed). Sem Liver Dis 1987; 7 (1).
7. Ross DS, *et al*. Am J Med 1983; 74: 464.
8. Schussler GC, *et al*. New Engl J Med 1978; 299: 510.
9. Janni A, *et al*. The Endocrines and the Liver (Langer M *et al*., Eds). London: Academic Press, 1983: 232.
10. Crowe J, *et al*. Gastroenterology 1980; 78: 1437.
11. Bannister P, *et al*. Ann Clin Biochem 1988; 25: 373.
12. Creutzfeldt W, *et al*. In: Falk Symposium 35 (Bianchi L *et al*., Eds). Lancaster: MTP Press Ltd, 1983: 221.
13. Prietto J, *et al*. Clin Endocrinol 1984; 21: 657.
14. Dymock IW, *et al*. Am J Med 1972; 52: 203.
15. Long RG, *et al*. Gut 1978; 19: 85.
16. Stellon AJ, *et al*. Gastroenterology 1985; 89: 1078.
17. Rees LH, *et al*. Lancet 1977; i: 726.

Suggested further reading

Bannister P and Losowsky MS. Sex hormones and chronic liver disease. J Hepatol 1988; 6: 258–262.

Chopra IJ, Solomon DH, Chopra U *et al*. Alterations in circulating thyroid hormones and thyrotropin in hepatic cirrhosis: evidence of euthyroidism despite subnormal serum triiodothyronine. J Clin Endocrinol Metab 1974; 39: 501–511.

Creutzfeldt W, Hartman H, Nauck M. *et al*. Liver disease and glucose homeostasis. In: Falk Symposium 35 (Bianchi L *et al*., Eds) Lancaster: MTP Press, 1983; 221–234.

Johnson PJ. Sex hormones and the liver. Clin Sci 1984; 66: 369–376.

Petrides AS and DeFronzo RA. Glucose and insulin metabolism in cirrhosis. J Hepatol 1989; 8: 107–114.

Van Thiel DH (Ed). Effects of pregnancy and sex hormones on the liver. Sem Liver Dios 1987; 7: (1).

8

Tumour markers

8.1 Introduction

Until recently, the diagnosis of cancer was based almost exclusively on the physical properties of the tumour. Some form of visual inspection of the tissue involved was required, either macroscopic (at operation or by use of an imaging technique) or microscopic. This approach has obvious limitations, in particular it is often difficult to locate the tumour precisely and it may be even more difficult to gain access to it.

A simple serological test which allows confident diagnosis and accurate monitoring of therapy has been a long-sought dream of the oncologist and the knowledge that some tumours synthesize and secrete substances (usually proteins) that show some degree of specificity for particular types of tumour has led to considerable research aimed at identifying such markers and applying them to clinical practice.

The ideal tumour marker would be one that is: (i) easily and reliably detected in serum, (ii) specific to a certain histological type of tumour, (iii) sufficiently sensitive to detect all cases of that tumour, (iv) detectable at a stage when the tumour is treatable, and (v) present in the serum at a concentration that is proportional to the viable tumour cell mass. This last criterion is particularly important if the test is to be of any value for monitoring therapy. To date, no such perfect test has been devised for any tumour, but in primary liver-cell carcinoma (hepatocellular carcinoma) one marker, α-fetoprotein, approaches the ideal.

8.2 Liver tumours

Like all tumours, those of the liver may be classified as benign or malignant, the latter being further sub-classified as primary or secondary. Primary hepatic tumours may arise from any of the cell types in the liver: *hepatocellular carcinoma* (HCC) from the hepatocytes, *cholangiocarcinoma* from the bile-duct cells, or *hepatic sarcoma* from the endothelial cells. In addition, the liver is the commonest site for secondary tumours which may originate from primary tumours of virtually any organ in the body.

In the West, primary liver cancer is relatively rare and patients with secondary hepatic malignancy outnumber those with primary tumours by about 50 : 1. In parts of sub-Saharan Africa and in the Middle and Far East, however, primary hepatocellular carcinoma is very common. It is a highly malignant tumour and patients seldom survive more than one year from the onset of symptoms. The wide geographical variation in the incidence of HCC is probably related to differences in the prevalence of hepatitis-B virus carriage in various countries (Chapter 5), for this together with chronic liver disease (and particularly cirrhosis) are the main aetiological factors in the development of HCC.

Diagnosis of HCC and other hepatic malignancies may be assisted by detection of one or other of the serum markers described below and/or the use of complementary diagnostic procedures including imaging techniques (to define the anatomical distribution of the tumour) and histological examination of biopsy specimens to confirm the histiogenesis. With the exception of carcinoembryonic antigen (Section 8.5.1), none of these tumour markers is of value in the diagnosis of secondary hepatic malignancy and the following discussion is therefore concerned essentially with markers of hepatocellular carcinoma.

8.3   α-Fetoprotein

α-Fetoprotein (AFP) is by far the most important serological tumour marker in hepatology [1]. It is a glycopeptide with a molecular weight of about 72 000 daltons comprised of 590 amino acids and a complex arrangement of carbohydrate side chains. It exists in several isoforms which differ with respect to their carbohydrate moieties and which may prove to be useful diagnostically (Section 8.3.6). AFP was first detected in 1963 in mice with chemically-induced liver tumours [2] and in a patient with HCC the following year [3], and was defined as an oncofetal protein. It has no known specific function but it shares many characteristics with albumin (with which it shows an overall sequence homology of about 40%) and of which it may be considered the embryonic analogue (by analogy with the foetal−adult haemoglobin system).

In the foetus, AFP is normally synthesized in large amounts only by the yolk sac, liver and gut. By the third month of gestation, foetal serum concentrations of AFP rise to levels of $2000-3000 \, \text{ng ml}^{-1}$ and, thereafter, fall progressively as albumin synthesis proceeds and the volume of distribution increases. Serum concentrations at one month after birth are about $30 \, \text{ng ml}^{-1}$ and the normal adult level of $2-5 \, \text{ng ml}^{-1}$ is reached by about one year of life [4] while, in the mother, serum AFP concentrations rise from about $30 \, \text{ng ml}^{-1}$ at 16 weeks gestation to $500 \, \text{ng ml}^{-1}$ at term (Fig. 8.1). In HCC, AFP

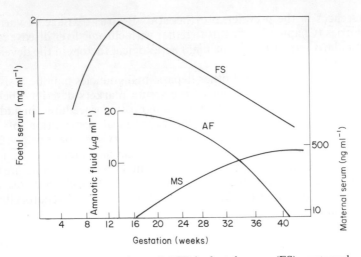

FIG. 8.1 Concentrations of AFP in foetal serum (FS), maternal serum (MS), and amniotic fluid (AF) in relation to gestational age (adapted from Lau and Larkins [4]).

appears to be synthesized solely by the malignant cells, because there is no evidence for reactive synthesis by surrounding non-malignant hepatocytes.

8.3.1 Detection of serum α-fetoprotein

Early studies in the 1970s used a simple immunodiffusion technique (see Section 6.9.1) with specific polyclonal antisera to detect AFP. Although this method was quite specific, it was not very sensitive and was able to detect AFP in serum only at concentrations exceeding 1000 ng ml^{-1} (Fig. 8.2) and it has largely been superseded by the very much more sensitive radioimmunoassays (RIAs) or enzyme-linked immunosorbent assays (ELISAs).

It is important to appreciate that the range of serum AFP concentrations encountered in clinical practice is very large indeed, i.e. from < 5 ng ml^{-1} in some normal subjects up to 10 000 000 ng ml^{-1} (10 g l^{-1}) in HCC patients (Fig. 8.2), and that the diagnostic significance of serum AFP is strongly related to its actual concentration. Many laboratories in which AFP measurements are performed mainly in the course of antenatal screening for the diagnosis of foetal neural

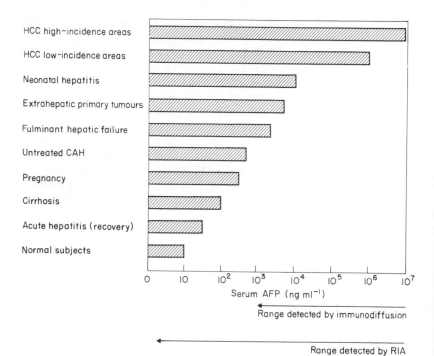

FIG. 8.2 Expected range of AFP in various disease states and pregnancy. It is apparent that an elevated serum AFP detected by immunodiffusion is highly specific for HCC, but equally many cases will be missed.

tube defects will have their assay systems adjusted to read accurately within the concentration range of 0–500 ng ml^{-1} (values above 500 ng ml^{-1} being rarely seen in pregnancy). Higher serum concentrations will be reported simply as >500 ng ml^{-1}, which is inadequate information in the context of hepatic malignancy. *It is therefore very important that the laboratory is informed when a diagnosis of HCC is suspected, so that the serum sample can be appropriately diluted to determine the precise concentration.*

8.3.2 Diagnosis of HCC in the symptomatic patient

When the more sensitive methods of detection are used (Section 8.3.1), serum AFP concentrations are found to be elevated above the reference range $(0-10 \text{ ng ml}^{-1})$ in about 80% of patients with symptomatic HCC overall, but are only occasionally increased in patients with metastatic liver disease and are almost always normal in those with other types of primary hepatic tumours. However, this frequency falls to about 50% in patients with HCC who do not have cirrhosis (Fig. 8.3). The interpretation of serum AFP results and their diagnostic value will therefore depend on the precise context in which they are being used.

For example, it is often necessary to determine whether clinical deterioration (e.g. accumulation of ascites) in a patient with cirrhosis is attributable to the development of HCC. In our experience, a serum AFP value of greater than 500 ng ml^{-1} is virtually diagnostic of HCC in this situation. A value between 10 and 500 ng ml^{-1} is, however, a grey area into which other non-malignant liver conditions may occasionally fall (see discussion of false-positive/negative results in Section 8.3.4).

A second situation in which AFP measurement can be useful is in determining whether, in a non-cirrhotic patient with suspected hepatic malignancy, the tumour is primary or secondary (a common clinical problem). Here, the serum AFP is somewhat less reliable. An elevated AFP above 1000 ng ml^{-1} will positively diagnose a primary tumour

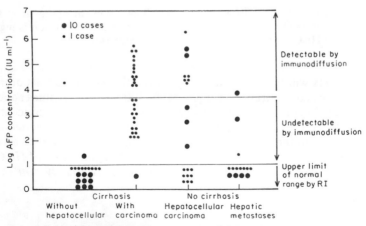

FIG. 8.3   Serum AFP levels used (i) to diagnose HCC in patients known to have cirrhosis and (ii) to differentiate between primary and secondary tumours of the liver. There is much less overlap in the former.

but, because only about 50% of such patients will have raised AFP levels, a negative result provides little information. Also, an AFP concentration between 10 and 1000 ng ml^{-1} in this situation may be misleading since such values can be found in some patients with secondary hepatic tumours and in other (non-malignant) liver conditions (see Fig. 8.2). Thus, only levels in excess of 1000 ng ml^{-1} should be taken as strong evidence of HCC in a patient known to have a tumour in a non-cirrhotic liver.

8.3.3 Screening for HCC in the asymptomatic patient

Despite the high specificity of a markedly elevated serum AFP concentration for HCC, it is really not worthwhile (on clinical or economic grounds) to screen large populations of patients who are at low risk of developing this tumour. It may, however, be more fruitful to screen high-risk groups (such as hepatitis B virus carriers or patients with cirrhosis) in whom the HCC detection rate will be about 5 per 1000 patients tested.

As noted above, the finding of an AFP concentration of > 500 ng ml^{-1} in a cirrhotic patient is virtually diagnostic of HCC, i.e. the specificity approaches 100%. A value between 50 and 500 ng ml^{-1} warrants more detailed investigation, both by repeating the test and by a radiological imaging technique. If a value between 10 and 50 ng ml^{-1} is obtained, the test should be repeated after three months (see Section 8.3.4).

There is no doubt that, if patients with cirrhosis are regularly screened at intervals of three to six months, a diagnosis of HCC can be established many months (and even years) before clinical symptoms develop. Whether or not this is of advantage to the patient is another matter. In the West, it is seldom feasible to resect the tumour in a cirrhotic liver, but there is some preliminary evidence that liver transplantation may be more successful (i.e. there is less chance of tumour recurrence) in patients in whom the diagnosis is established before clinical symptoms develop.

In high-incidence areas, particularly China, other parts of the Far East and in Alaska, where HCC is very common, mass screening programmes for elevated serum AFP concentrations (usually coupled with ultrasound scanning) have been instituted and have led to the early detection of tumours [5]. It appears that, in these countries, the tumour develops when the cirrhosis is at a less advanced stage and is often resectable and evidence from China suggests that screening programmes are beginning to have a real impact on survival. The AFP levels seen in patients with these smaller, presymptomatic tumours are generally lower than in symptomatic patients. Data from Japan [6] show that serum AFP concentrations above $400\,\text{ng}\,\text{ml}^{-1}$ are seen in only 25% of patients with tumours smaller than 3 cm, compared with 60% of those with larger tumours.

8.3.4 False-positive results

In view of the increasing use of serum AFP in the diagnosis of HCC, it is important to be aware that there are several other hepatic conditions in which levels above the reference range of $0-10\,\text{ng}\,\text{ml}^{-1}$ may be found. Patients with uncomplicated cirrhosis may occasionally have serum AFP concentrations up to $100\,\text{ng}\,\text{ml}^{-1}$ without any evidence of HCC and those with untreated chronic active hepatitis (with or without cirrhosis) can, also occasionally, have levels as high as $500\,\text{ng}\,\text{ml}^{-1}$. This presents a major diagnostic problem because the presence of a complicating HCC is a real possibility. In these situations, the recommendation is to repeat the measurement of serum AFP at three-month intervals to determine whether its concentration is rising (see Sections 8.3.6 and 8.4).

Other conditions in which elevated serum concentrations of AFP are found include fulminant hepatic failure, in which the AFP is often raised (occasionally as high as $1000\,\text{ng}\,\text{ml}^{-1}$). Minor elevations of AFP are also often seen in the later stages of uncomplicated acute viral hepatitis but concentrations rarely exceed $100\,\text{ng}\,\text{ml}^{-1}$. Neither of these conditions should cause any diagnostic confusion, for HCC does not usually enter the differential diagnosis of patients presenting with hepatitic illnesses. However, it should be noted that up to 5% of primary tumours other than HCC secrete AFP. This is particularly the case with tumours of the pancreas, stomach and gall-bladder, and metastases therefrom to the liver, but serum AFP concentrations seldom exceed $1000\,\text{ng}\,\text{ml}^{-1}$.

In some of the above conditions it would appear that the minor elevations in serum AFP concentration may be related to hepatocellular regeneration and, indeed, the role of AFP as an indicator of regeneration is the subject of much current research. Interpretation of these minor increases in AFP levels in terms of regeneration is, however, very complex because following partial hepatectomy (when there is the most intense hepatic regeneration) there is no change in serum AFP concentration.

8.3.5 False-negative results

Overall, about 20% of cases of HCC have serum AFP concentrations that fall within the normal reference range. This is particularly so in that minority of patients who do not have an underlying cirrhosis, up to half of whom may have AFP levels of less than $10 \, \text{ng ml}^{-1}$. Further screening for AFP in these cases is of no value, because if a particular tumour does not secrete AFP at presentation it will not do so during the subsequent course of the disease, i.e. AFP-negative tumours do not become AFP-positive tumours (nor *vice versa*). In these cases, other tumour markers (see below) may be evaluated.

8.3.6 Improving the specificity of serum AFP

As noted above (Section 8.3.2), the range of serum AFP concentrations between 10 and $500 \, \text{ng ml}^{-1}$ constitutes a grey area for interpretation. A value within this range, obtained from a single measurement of serum AFP, is not very specific for HCC. The specificity can, however, be improved by serial testing. Thus, patients with HCC will show a steady rise in serum AFP (which may not necessarily exceed $500 \, \text{ng ml}^{-1}$) over the space of a few months, whereas those without HCC show fluctuating levels or, in the case of chronic active hepatitis treated with corticosteroids, the serum concentrations fall to within the normal range when the disease becomes less active.

An alternative approach that may prove useful is based on recent evidence that there appear to be several isoforms of AFP that differ from each other mainly with respect to the composition of their carbohydrate side chains and that these can be distinguished by differential binding to various plant lectins on affinity columns (Table 8.1). Thus, the carbohydrate side chain of serum AFP derived from HCC binds strongly to both Concanavalin A (Con A) and to lentil lectins, while AFP from cirrhotic patients without HCC binds

TABLE 8.1 Binding of serum AFP to plant lectins

Serum AFP from	Binding to concanavilin A	Binding to lentil lectins
Hepatocellular carcinoma (HCC)	+ + +	+ + +
Cirrhosis (without HCC)	+ + +	+
Metastases	+	+ + +

similarly to Con-A but only weakly to lentil lectins and serum AFP produced by secondary liver tumours binds strongly to the lentil lectins but only weakly to Con-A [6].

These differences are attributable to the presence or absence of N-acetyl-glucosamine, mannose and glucose (in the case of Con-A binding) and fucose (in the case of lentil lectin binding) in the different isoforms of AFP. This analytical approach is potentially very useful for differential diagnosis, particularly during screening programmes when moderately elevated serum AFP concentrations are frequently found, but absolute values for binding to the affinity columns vary between laboratories and consensus figures are not yet available.

8.4 Role of serum AFP in the management of HCC

Serial AFP measurements can be extremely useful for monitoring responses to treatment (chemotherapy, resection, arterial emboliza-tion or transplantation) in patients with AFP-positive HCC. For a given patient, the serum AFP concentration usually behaves as if it is proportional to the total tumour mass and will increase exponentially (with a doubling time of approximately 40 days [7]) in the absence of treatment, but will also decrease in proportion to remaining viable tumour mass when effective treatment is instituted. With surgical removal of the tumour (either by resection or by liver transplanta-tion), serum AFP concentrations fall to within the normal range with a half-life of about four days. It should be noted, however, that a fall in AFP level to within the normal range following resection does not necessarily imply that all of the tumour has been removed. It seems that there is a minimum threshold mass of tumour that is required to produce sufficient AFP to lift the serum concentration above the normal range (Fig. 8.4) and small amounts of residual tumour may be insufficient to give an increased serum AFP. In this situation the serum AFP level should be monitored monthly for several months to determine whether it is rising again, which indicates regrowth of the tumour.

The fall in serum AFP concentrations following effective chemo-therapy can be exploited for the *in vivo* testing of anti-cancer drugs. Following the institution of a course of treatment with a particular drug, a decrease in serum AFP levels during the subsequent one or two

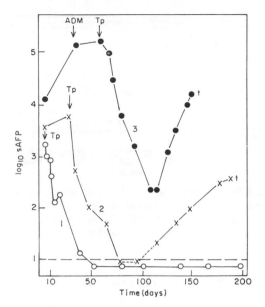

FIG. 8.4 Changes in AFP following orthotopic liver transplantation for HCC. There was no macroscopic evidence of tumour after operation in any patient. Patient 1 remains well 10 years after transplantation. Patient 2 showed subsequent recurrence despite having achieved normal AFP levels. Patient 3 did not achieve normal AFP levels at any time suggesting residual microscopic tumour deposits.

months indicates that the drug is effective and should be continued (Fig. 8.5). A continued rise in serum AFP indicates that the tumour is resistant and another drug should be tried if this is deemed appropriate. This approach avoids prolonged (potentially toxic) chemotherapy in patients who will not benefit from it.

It should be noted that, while there is no direct relationship between serum AFP (either its presence or absence or absolute concentrations) and prognosis, patients with normal or only slowly rising serum AFP concentrations tend to survive longer. Patients with relentlessly increasing serum AFP levels despite one or more courses of chemotherapy have a poor prognosis.

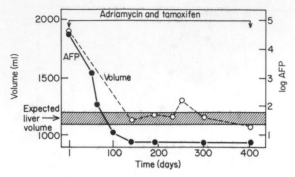

FIG. 8.5 Changes in AFP following cytotoxic chemotherapy. This patient underwent complete clinical remission. Serum AFP levels fell in parallel with the decreasing liver volume as measured by ultrasound examination.

8.4.1 Serum AFP in paediatric practice

Grossly elevated serum AFP concentrations are seen in virtually all children with hepatoblastoma and in about 75% with hepatocellular carcinoma. However, neonatal hepatitis of any cause is also associated with abnormal serum AFP levels and this renders AFP of little diagnostic value during the first year of life. Other childhood disorders in which high serum AFP concentrations may be found include tyrosinaemia and the ataxiatelangiectasia syndrome.

8.5 Other serum markers of hepatocellular carcinoma

The extent to which other tumour markers are used depends on the prevalence of the HCC in the population served by a particular laboratory. In the UK and in other Western countries (where HCC is not a major clinical problem), the only tumour markers (apart from AFP) for which testing services are widely available are the so-called hepatoma alkaline phosphatase (H-ALP), serum ferritin and carcinoembryonic antigen (CEA). The latter two are not of particular diagnostic value because the serum levels seem to reflect underlying liver disease rather than the tumour itself. In addition, CEA is not specific for liver tumours and serum ferritin concentrations are elevated in a number of quite specific conditions in the absence of hepatic malignancy (see Chapter 11).

Other serum markers of HCC that have been defined include a hepatoma-specific gamma-glutamyltranspeptidase and des-gamma-carboxy prothrombin. It should be stressed that, by comparison with AFP, experience with these other markers is limited. It is characteristic of newly described tumour markers that, while they usually perform well under clinical study conditions where the numbers of patients with the "index" condition and the various control groups are similar, they tend to perform less well in routine clinical practice where patients with the index condition are outnumbered 100 : 1 (or, in screening studies, by several thousands to one) by those without the condition. Nevertheless, these additional markers are fairly widely used in countries where HCC is a major problem, particularly in Japan.

In addition to the above, there have been several reports of inappropriate secretion of various hormones by HCC and each of these could, in theory, be used as a tumour marker, particularly for monitoring response to therapy. These are dealt with in some detail in Chapter 7.

8.5.1 Hepatoma-specific alkaline phosphatase

Hepatoma-specific alkaline phosphatase (H-ALP) is an isoenzyme of alkaline phosphatase (ALP); it is also sometimes known as variant ALP [8]. It has properties akin to those of foetal intestinal ALP and is highly specific for HCC, false-positive results being most unusual. However, it occurs in only about 30% of cases from areas where there is a high incidence of HCC and in less than 5% of those from low-incidence areas.

H-ALP can be detected by the same routine gel electrophoresis procedures used to identify other ALP isoenzymes (Chapter 2) and is identified as a fast-moving band running ahead of the main liver band (Fig. 8.6). H-ALP can be further distinguished from normal ALP by the fact that it has a lower molecular weight, is less sensitive to inhibition by L-phenylalanine and is less retarded on gel electrophoresis after treatment with neuraminidase. In addition, H-ALP is quite distinct from the placental isoenzyme (biochemically identical to the Regan isoenzyme) which is detectable in the sera of up to 10% of patients with various primary non-hepatic tumours.

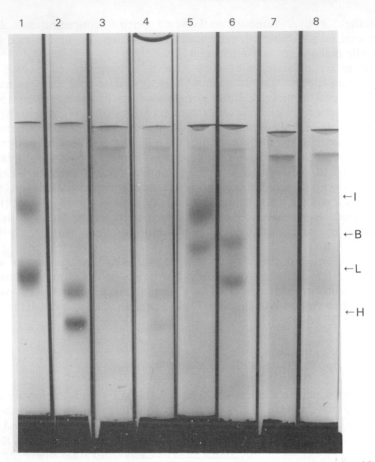

FIG. 8.6 Electrophoresis of alkaline phosphatase on polyacrylamide gels from six patients with liver disease. The three normal bands (I = intestine, B = bone and L = liver) which are of variable intensity are marked. In gels 2, 3 and 4, particularly 2, additional bands are seen – the so-called hepatoma isoenzymes (H). All these patients did in fact have histological confirmation of hepatocellular carcinoma.

8.5.2 Hepatoma specific gamma-glutamyltranspeptidase

Serum from patients with hepatobiliary disease, when electrophoresed on polyacrylamide gradient gels, gives up to 13 bands that stain for gamma-glutamyltranspeptidase (GGTP). Three of these bands, II, II′ and I′, appear to be highly specific for HCC and at least one is detectable in about 50% of patients with HCC compared with less than 5% of those with other hepatobiliary disorders [9].

The basis of the differences between the various bands, as is the case with H-ALP and AFP (at least partly), lies in the carbohydrate side-chain compositions. It is therefore interesting that the activity of α-L-fucosidase, a lysosomal enzyme which catabolizes fucoproteins and may reflect increased fucose turnover in malignant tissue, has been found to be elevated in the serum of 75% of patients with HCC [10]. Reactivation of other foetal enzymes which are involved in the modification of the carbohydrate side chains of glycoproteins during processing and secretion from the hepatocyte may also be involved. All of the tests based on detection of isoenzymes show considerable potential, but their application is limited by the laborious methodology. The development of simpler immunoassay systems using specific antisera to the various isoenzymes is proving difficult. A radioimmunoassay for HCC-derived GGTP has recently been reported and appears to be useful in distinguishing HCC from non-malignant chronic liver diseases, but a high frequency of this marker was also found in other primary liver tumours and in metastatic liver disease.

8.5.3 Des-gamma-carboxy prothrombin

When blood levels of vitamin K are low, the decreased activity of vitamin K dependent prothrombin carboxylase results in the release of an abnormal prothrombin, des-gamma-carboxy prothrombin. High concentrations of this abnormal prothrombin have been reported in over 90% of patients with HCC and 70% of these had levels higher than $300 \, ng \, ml^{-1}$ [11]. In that study, only one of 17 patients with metastatic liver disease gave a positive result and all of 17 other patients with chronic hepatitis were negative. The specificity of the test may be improved by parenteral administration of vitamin K. In patients without HCC, this results in normalization of the des-gamma-carboxy prothrombin concentration, while in those with HCC there is a transient decrease followed by a return (within two weeks) to the initial elevated levels [12].

8.5.4 Tumour markers in fibrolamellar carcinoma

The rare histological variant of hepatocellular carcinoma, fibrolamellar carcinoma, is associated with two serum markers that may be useful in diagnosis and management: the *unsaturated vitamin B_{12} binding capacity* and *neurotensin*, both of which are grossly elevated. It is important to establish the diagnosis of fibrolamellar carcinoma when it occurs, for the prognosis and the frequency with which successful resection can be performed is much better than for other types of HCC.

8.6 Tumour markers in secondary liver cancer

Tumour markers are of far less importance in the diagnosis and management of the more common liver tumours that originate from primary tumours elsewhere. With the notable exception of markers related to carcinoid tumours (see Section 8.7), CEA is the only serum marker that is of proven value in secondary liver cancer.

8.6.1 Carcinoembryonic antigen

Carcinoembryonic antigen (CEA) was first described by Gold and Freeman in 1965 [13] and was the first tumour marker of any kind to be widely used clinically. The antigen was derived from colonic carcinoma tissue and initial experience, using relatively insensitive assays, suggested that a positive serum test was diagnostic of colonic carcinoma. However, with the advent of more sensitive assays, it became apparent that CEA is present at low levels in normal serum and at higher concentrations in patients with non-colonic primary tumours as well as in patients with benign colonic disorders.

CEA is a glycoprotein with a molecular weight of 200 000 which is synthesized in small amounts by the normal gut but is produced in much greater quantities by colorectal carcinomas. The amount synthesized varies greatly from one tumour to the next and serum concentrations will also depend on the vascularity of the particular tumour. CEA is cleared by the liver, being desialylated (probably by Kupffer cells) and then removed by hepatocytes through a receptor-mediated endocytotic mechanism involving binding to the asialo-glycoprotein receptor (see Chapter 6) via terminal galactose residues on the asialo-CEA that have been exposed by the desialylation. It is therefore perhaps unsurprising that high serum CEA concentrations are found in several benign hepatic conditions [14], including cirrhosis, biliary-tract obstruction and hepatic metastases [15], where this mechanism of clearance may be impaired. Partly because of this, CEA is no longer widely used as a diagnostic test for colonic carcinoma either in the symptomatic patient or for screening high-risk populations.

From a hepatological point of view, the major role for CEA lies in the detection of hepatic metastases in patients who have undergone attempted curative resection of colonic primary tumours [16]. Rapidly rising concentrations, where levels of greater than 40 ng ml^{-1} are reached within six months of the first detection of seropositivity, are strongly suggestive of liver metastases. Such changes often predate clinical symptoms by up to six months (Fig. 8.7) and presumably reflect both the ease of secretion into the blood of CEA produced in the liver and possible diminished clearance as a consequence of hepatocellular damage related to the developing metastases. Several groups of workers are now actively assessing the value of further laparotomy in patients showing rising CEA levels, with a view to resection of recurrent disease which may be visible at operation but may still be asymptomatic. Serum CEA is much less useful for detecting local recurrence of tumour (Table 8.2), but a fall in serum concentration following intra-arterial chemotherapy predicts subsequent clinical response [17].

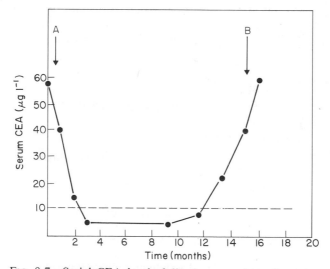

Fig. 8.7 Serial CEA levels following resection of a colonic carcinoma. There was no evidence of hepatic deposits at the time of the initial resection (A), but hepatic tumour could be detected on CT scanning at time B, four months after the CEA level started to rise.

TABLE 8.2   Correlation of carcinoembryonic antigen levels with pattern of recurrent colorectal cancer: liver metastases are associated with high CEA levels, local recurrence with low levels (adapted from Wanebo *et al.* [16]).

Site of recurrence	No. of patients	Level (ng ml^{-1})					
		0–2·5	2·6–5·0	5–10	10·1–20	> 20	> 100
Liver only	52	4	0	2	6	15	25
Local	46	17	6	6	7	9	1

8.7   Carcinoid tumours and the carcinoid syndrome

Carcinoid tumours are derived from enterochromaffin (Kulchintzky) cells, which are widely distributed throughout the body. Those tumours that originate in the small bowel often produce large quantities of vasoactive peptides, most notably *serotonin*. This is inactivated by the liver until hepatic metastases develop, whereupon serotonin is released into the systemic circulation and causes the *carcinoid syndrome* of episodic flushing and diarrhoea.

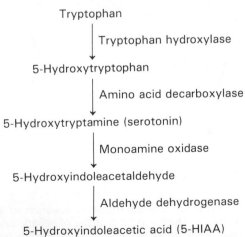

FIG. 8.8   Pathway of 5-HIAA production in the carcinoid syndrome.

Detection of one of the metabolites of serotonin in the urine is a most valuable test for the diagnosis of this condition and for monitoring therapy. The metabolite of choice is 5-hydroxyindole acetic acid (5-HIAA), which is the final product of the metabolic pathway (Fig. 8.8). Normally, less than 10 mg of 5-HIAA is excreted in the urine in 24 h and a level of greater than 30 mg per 24 h is considered virtually diagnostic of carcinoid. False-negative results occur with foregut tumours, which often lack the amino acid decarboxylase and consequently secrete 5-hydroxytryptophan rather than serotonin. On the other hand, false-positive results can be obtained in patients taking drugs such as methysergide (widely used in the treatment of carcinoid syndrome) or those who have eaten foods such as bananas, pineapples, walnuts or avocados, which are rich in serotonin. The level of 5-HIAA in a 24-h urine collection reflects tumour mass and offers a useful method of monitoring the effects of treatment, the most widely used approach to which is occlusion of the hepatic artery either by embolization or ligation (Fig. 8.9).

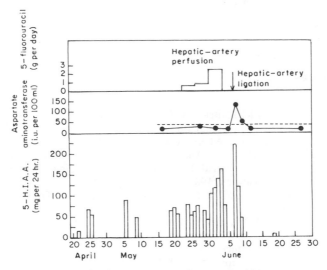

FIG. 8.9 Monitoring response of a carcinoid tumour to treatment using serial monitoring of 24-hour urinary 5-HIAA. There was no response to hepatic artery perfusion of the cytotoxic drug 5-fluorouracil, but hepatic artery ligation led to a fall in urinary 5-HIAA to undetectable levels. Note the transient rise in AST reflecting tumour necrosis. The patient lost all symptoms.

8.8 Liver function tests in hepatic malignancy

Apart from the fact that hepatic malignancy can be virtually excluded if the serum activities of the liver enzymes (AST, ALT, ALP, GGPT and 5-NT) are within their normal ranges, the routine liver-function tests are of little value in the diagnosis of liver tumours because there are so many other causes of abnormalities in these tests that a positive diagnosis cannot be established with any confidence. Serial changes may be more informative and, as previously noted, an unexplained steady rise in ALP is particularly indicative of a space-occupying lesion, particularly if the serum bilirubin concentration is normal. In patients with hepatic tumours, the serum bilirubin does not usually begin to rise until the terminal stages, unless there is additional underlying chronic liver disease or tumour deposits occlude bile ducts and cause obstruction. However, rising ALP activities must not be considered diagnostic of hepatic malignancy because similar changes are common in other conditions (see especially Chapter 12).

References

1. Wespic HT and Kirkpatrick A. Gastroenterology 1979; 77: 787.
2. Abelev GI *et al*. Transplant Bull 1963; 1: 174.
3. Tartarinov YS. Vor Med Klin (Mosc) 1964; 10: 90.
4. Lau HL and Larkins SE. Am J Obstet Gynaecol 1976; 124: 533.
5. Tang ZY. In: Subclinical Hepatocellular Carcinoma. Beijing: China Academic Publications, 1985: 1–11.
6. Sawabu N and Hattori N. In: Neoplasms of the Liver. Tokyo: Springer-Verlag, 1987: 227–237.
7. Johnson PJ and Williams R. J Natl Cancer Inst 1980; 64: 1329.
8. Suzuki H *et al*. Ann NY Acad Sci 1975; 259: 307.
9. Sawubo N *et al*. Cancer 1983; 51: 327.
10. Deugnier Y *et al*. Hepatology 1984; 4: 889.
11. Liebmann HA *et al*. N Engl J Med 1984; 310: 1427.
12. Lefrere J-J *et al*. J Hepatol 1987; 5: 27.
13. Gold P and Freeman SO. J Exp Med 1965; 121: 439.
14. Loewenstein MS, Zmachek N. Gastroenterology 1977; 72: 161.
15. Begent RHJ. Ann Clin Biochem 1984; 21: 231.
16. Wanebo WJ *et al*. N Engl J Med 1978; 299: 448.
17. Sears HJF *et al*. J Clin Oncol 1985; 8: 108.

Suggested further reading

Begent RHJ. The value of carcinoembryonic antigen measurement in clinical practice. Ann Clin Biochem 1984; 21: 231–238.

Maton PN and Hodgson HIF. Carcinoid tumours and the carcinoid syndrome. In: Textbook of Gastroenterology. (Bouchier IAD, Allen RN, Hodgson HSF and Keighley MRB, Eds). Eastbourne: Baillière Tindall, 1984: 620–634.

Sawabu N and Hattori N. Serological markers in hepatocellular carcinoma. In: Neoplasms of the Liver (Okuda K and Ishak KG, Eds). Tokyo: Springer-Verlag, 1987.

Warnes TW and Smith A. Tumour markers in diagnosis and management. In: Liver Tumours (Johnson PJ and Williams R, Eds). Baillière's Clinical Gastroenterology, 1981: 1.

9

Drugs and other chemical hepatotoxins

9.1 Introduction

The list of drugs and other chemical agents that can cause liver damage increases year by year and is now very long indeed. To cover adequately all these agents and the various mechanisms involved is beyond the scope of this book and this chapter is intended only as an *aide mémoire* to the possibility that an abnormal liver function test (LFT) may be drug-related. For more detailed information, any one of the many excellent texts on this subject may be consulted (see, Suggested Further Reading).

9.2 Mechanisms of chemical hepatotoxicity

Most drugs and many other potentially toxic chemicals are metabolized by the liver and, partly because of its central role in this respect and partly because it is the organ that usually receives the largest initial dose of xenobiotics (drugs and other foreign chemicals) taken orally, it is particularly susceptible to damage by chemical agents. Overall, the biochemical reactions involved in drug metabolism by the liver result in detoxification by conversion of the relatively non-polar (lipid-soluble) compounds into polar (water-soluble) substances which can then be excreted in the bile or the urine. These reactions are catalysed by a large number of enzymes but the most quantitatively important are those comprising the mixed-function oxidase system (MFOS).

Most of the enzymes involved in drug metabolism exist as families of related isoenzymes (e.g. the cytochromes P-450), each with discrete but overlapping substrate specificities capable of handling a broad range of both xenobiotics and endogenous compounds. Thus, competition between endogenous substances and exogenous compounds (e.g. drugs) can lead to unexpected toxicity. The same pathways can sometimes lead to production of reactive metabolites which readily bind to various cellular macromolecules such as nucleic acids and proteins and can cause neoplastic changes or cell death. In addition, each of the drug metabolizing enzyme systems is under homeostatic control influenced by genetic and environmental factors and several of these systems show reduced activity in the neonate and sometimes also in the elderly and the consequent deficient metabolism can lead to direct toxicity through the pharmacological effects of the parent drug.

Other factors that can diminish enzyme activity, and thereby enhance chemical hepatotoxicity, include malnutrition (especially protein deficiency) and severe disease. This is particularly true of liver disease, in which the decreased overall metabolic activity of the damaged organ, its decreased synthetic function (with consequent hypoalbuminaemia, leading to reduction in protein binding and increased concentrations of the free drug in the circulation), and extrahepatic shunting (which will alter blood flow and delivery of the chemical agent to the liver; see Section 1.3.1), can profoundly affect the hepatotoxicity of xenobiotics.

9.2.1 Enzyme induction and inhibition

Many substances are capable of stimulating (inducing) synthesis of the enzymes involved in their own metabolism. From the point of drug toxicity this can be either advantageous or disadvantageous. If it is the parent compound that is toxic, enzyme induction can lead to a higher rate of conversion to non-toxic metabolites and thus increase tolerance for the drug. On the other hand, if a metabolite of the drug is the toxic agent, enzyme induction may increase production of the toxic metabolite.

In many instances, these effects are predictable and therapeutic dosages of drugs are set at levels which take account of them. A problem arises, however, when two or more drugs or other chemical agents handled by the same enzyme system are taken simultaneously. If a metabolite of one of these is toxic and the other drug is an inducing agent, the second can increase the toxic effects of the first. Alternatively, the inducer may enhance elimination of the other drug, necessitating administration of a higher dose to obtain the required therapeutic effect and *vice versa* upon withdrawal of the inducing agent.

Conversely, many xenobiotics can inhibit (competitively) or inactivate (e.g. by formation of enzyme–drug complexes) one or more preformed enzymes along the detoxification pathways, resulting in elevated blood or tissue concentrations of the agents and/or their metabolites. Thus, even if a particular inhibitor is itself relatively non-toxic, it can considerably increase the toxicity of other agents taken concurrently.

9.3 Classification of hepatotoxic agents

Several systems of classification and cross-classification of hepatotoxic chemicals have been adopted by various authors over the years according to which viewpoint of hepatotoxicity is being presented. The following are some of the more commonly used systems.

9.3.1 Predictable/idiosyncratic hepatotoxins

A *predictable* (sometimes termed intrinsic) hepatotoxin is one which produces liver damage (in humans and/or experimental animals) in a high proportion of individuals and in a dose-related manner. An *idiosyncratic* toxin causes liver damage in only a small proportion of individuals exposed to the agent and in a manner which is usually not dose-dependent and which is difficult to reproduce in experimental animals. Idiosyncratic reactions usually manifest themselves within a short time after initial exposure to the agent (a few days or a few weeks) but have been noted in patients taking drugs for longer periods without any apparent side-effects. They may be due to genetic abnormalities, either in the individual's metabolism of the agent and/or that predispose to the development of a hypersensitivity state.

9.3.2 Direct/indirect hepatotoxins

Direct hepatotoxins are agents (or their metabolites) that exert direct physico-chemical actions (e.g. denaturation of proteins, lipid peroxidation) which alter and disrupt cellular organelles. *Indirect* toxins are those which act as antimetabolites, interfering with some vital metabolic process which then leads to a structural injury that is secondary to the metabolic lesion. Examples of the former include carbon tetrachloride, while the latter term covers a wide range of substances such as paracetamol (acetaminophen), ethanol and various antineoplastic drugs. Most of the direct and many of the indirect hepatotoxins are also predictable hepatotoxins.

9.3.3 Cholestatic/hepatocellular hepatotoxins

This classification is concerned with the site of action of the hepatotoxin and with the resulting biochemical abnormalities. It is particularly useful as a first step in diagnosis, because it can be employed to narrow down the range of possible toxic agents according to the pattern of abnormal LFTs and, for this reason, is used here. Its main disadvantage is the great deal of overlap in the system, for some "hepatocellular" lesions may be accompanied by cholestasis and, conversely, prolonged cholestasis often leads to at least some hepatocellular injury.

9.4 Diagnostic considerations

The diagnosis of chemically-induced hepatic injury can be very difficult, because the usual investigations (including liver biopsy) are seldom able to distinguish this from cholestasis or hepatitis due to other causes. In addition, the particular circumstances may themselves serve to confuse, for it is easy to attribute hepatic abnormalities to a hepatotoxic xenobiotic to which it is known the patient has been exposed when exposure to that agent may be only coincidental to liver disease of another aetiology. Conversely, the changes induced by many hepatotoxins are often indistinguishable from those associated with other liver disorders (see Table 9.1) and such agents may be overlooked as a cause of the hepatic injury.

A detailed history is essential and care must be taken to exclude all other causes of liver damage (Table 9.2). Thus, information must be obtained about travel to countries where infectious diseases of the liver are endemic and about contacts with others who may either have travelled to such areas or who actually have an infectious disorder. Parenteral exposure to blood products and occupational or environmental exposure to hepatotoxins (Section 9.19) must be documented. Since alcohol (Chapter 10) is an inducing agent [1] that can augment the liver-damaging potential of other compounds (Section 9.2.1), a precise drinking history should be obtained. Information must be elicited about all medications (whether prescribed or not) that the patient may have been taking, with careful attention to combinations of drugs that might act together (Section 9.2.1) to produce liver damage. Local homeopathic practices must be borne in mind, in areas where consumption of "bush teas" and other herbal infusions is common, the possibility should always be considered that components of such extracts may themselves be hepatotoxic (Section 9.18) or may act synergistically with more conventional therapeutic agents.

Finally, it is important to note that whereas many nations now have strict controls regulating the marketing of drugs and potentially hazardous chemicals, this is not universal. Some of the hepatotoxic agents to which reference is made here have now been withdrawn from use in Europe, North America and several other countries but are still available elsewhere.

TABLE 9.1. Examples of drugs which can induce liver damage with associated clinical, biochemical or histological features that may be confused with liver disorders of other aetiologies

Differential diagnosis	Cause of liver damage
Acute viral hepatitis	Benzodiazepines
	Phenytoin
	Halothane
	Iproniazid
	Isoniazid
	Methyldopa
	Nitrofurantoin
	p-Aminosalicylic acid
	Phenylbutazone
	Rifampicin
	Sodium valproate
	Sulphonamides
Autoimmune chronic active hepatitis	Aspirin
	Carbutamide
	Methyldopa
	Nitrofurantoin
	Phenylbutazone
	Thioureas
Extrahepatic biliary obstruction	C-17 Alkylated steroids
	Chlorpromazine
	Chlorpropamide
	Erythromycin estolate
	Rifampicin
Primary biliary cirrhosis	Ajmaline
	Chlorpromazine
	Thiobendazole
	Tolbutamide
Alcoholic liver disease	Amiodarone
	Methotrexate
	Perhexiline

TABLE 9.2.   Investigation of suspected chemically-induced liver damage

---

1. Document exposure
   (a) prescribed drugs
   (b) self-administered drugs/herbal products
   (c) occupational/environmental agents
   (d) alcohol
   (e) combinations of the above

2. Relate (1) to onset of illness/abnormality

3. Classify LFT abnormalities
   (a) Hyperbilirubinaemia alone, see Section 9.6
   (b) Two or more abnormal cholestatic indices, see Section 9.6
   (c) Predominantly hepatocellular, see Section 9.8
   (d) Mixed pattern, see Sections 9.6 and 9.7

4. Compare (3) with reported hepatotoxicity of agents identified in (1),
    see e.g. Tables 9.3 and 9.4

5. Exclude other causes
   (a) Microbial infection, see Chapters 5 and 12.
   (b) Immunological disorders, see Chapter 6.
   (c) Metabolic diseases, see Chapter 11.
   (d) Biliary disease (ultrasonography, cholecystography, etc.)
   (e) See also Table 9.1

6. Check haematological parameters against clinical findings, (e.g. eosino-
    philia with a rash, fever, etc., might suggest hypersensitivity to the
    suspected agent)

7. Observe effect of withdrawing suspected agent

8. Do not challenge (unless continued use of drug is absolutely essential,
    in which event re-introduce with extreme caution)

9.5 Laboratory investigations

Biochemical LFTs are widely used to screen for chemical hepatotoxicity because they are cheap, safe, simple to perform and are easily
repeatable. Furthermore, they are often the only abnormalities
detected, because there is frequently no clinical evidence of liver

damage, but they also comprise the first line of investigation when signs or symptoms do develop (see Chapter 2).

However, while the LFTs are of value in monitoring prolonged therapy with drugs that are known to be potentially hepatotoxic, they are of less use for detecting idiosyncratic reactions (Section 9.3.1) to drugs that do not usually damage the liver or which are given for short periods only. Also, many drugs can cause transient abnormalities that are of questionable significance and which may disappear despite continuation of the drug while, on the other hand, liver damage can occur without any test abnormality being detected (see Chapter 2).

It is, nevertheless, worthwhile to periodically check the biochemical LFTs of individuals who are on long-term medication with potentially hepatotoxic therapeutic agents and also of patients who fall into one of the susceptible groups with deficient drug-metabolizing capacity, e.g. neonates, the elderly, and those with known metabolic disorders. Patients with liver disease who are being treated (whether for their liver condition or for some concomitant disorder) with drugs that have a narrow therapeutic range should be carefully monitored. If, as a consequence of the liver disease, the prothrombin time is prolonged or the serum albumin falls below about 30 gl^{-1}, it can be assumed that there is impaired drug metabolism and particular caution should be exercised, for this can lead to increased (possibly toxic) blood levels of the drug in patients on a standard therapeutic dose (see Section 9.2).

If drug hepatotoxicity is suspected and an adequate history cannot be obtained, a comprehensive drug screen may be necessary, which will require the services of a specialized laboratory. In the final analysis, even if firm suspicion points to a particular drug or other chemical agent, proof may not be forthcoming without a challenge. However, *it is strongly recommended that challenge tests be avoided because of the risk of precipitating severe (possibly fatal) liver disease*. It is very rare that an alternative drug is not available when therapy is essential and challenges with suspected hepatotoxic agents should not be undertaken lightly.

9.6 Drug-induced hyperbilirubinaemia

Chemically-induced hyperbilirubinaemia, as the sole biochemical abnormality and of sufficient degree to produce jaundice, occurs rarely. Mild hyperbilirubinaemias (i.e. without jaundice), however, can frequently be drug-related.

Several therapeutic agents can produce *unconjugated hyper-bilirubinaemia* either by directly inducing haemolysis or by interfering with those aspects of transport of bilirubin from blood to bile that precede conjugation. Examples of the former include sulphasalazine, sulphonamides and methyldopa and, of the latter, some of the antimicrobials (e.g. rifampicin, novobiocin; Section 9.13) and other substances such as the cholecystographic agent *bunamiodyl*, which is no longer in general use.

Agents that interfere with later stages of bilirubin transport and excretion into bile give rise to *conjugated hyperbilirubinaemia*. Many plant alkaloids, a classical example of which is *icterogenin* (derived from the plant *Lippia rhemani*), and the C-17 alkylated steroids and related compounds (Section 9.16) fall into this category.

9.7 Cholestatic liver injury

Potentially, the more serious of the chemically-induced hyper-bilirubinaemias are those which are accompanied by mild to marked elevations in serum alkaline phosphatase (ALP) and gamma-glutamyl-transpeptidase (GGTP) activities. However, the GGTP is very sensitive to xenobiotics and can often be elevated on its own or when there are only mild increases in serum bilirubin concentrations and/or ALP activities. Whether this is actually a reflection of mild liver injury is often difficult to establish but it seems likely that in many such instances the increased GGTP may be due to a particular susceptibility of the enzyme for its synthesis to be increased by the action of inducing agents (Section 9.2.1), such as alcohol, and may not necessarily be an indication of liver-cell damage. This may also be the case with ALP, which can be elevated (with or without a concomitant rise in serum bilirubin or GGTP) in the absence of any overt liver damage, as is often seen, for example, in patients treated with anti-rheumatic drugs. In these situations, the serum biochemical abnormalities almost always show a rapid return to normality upon cessation of exposure to the causative agent. Examples of drugs that may cause a cholestatic pattern of LFT abnormalities are given in Table 9.3.

TABLE 9.3. Examples of drugs that can cause a predominantly cholestatic pattern of LFT abnormalities[a]

Ajmaline (M)	Nitrofurans
Anabolic steroids (C-17)	Oestradiol
Arsenicals	Penicillamine
Benzodiazepines (M)	Phenindione (M)
Carbimazole	Phenothiazines (M)
Cephalosporins	Saramycetin
Chlorpropamide	Sulphonamides
Cyclophosphamide	Thiabendazole
Cytosine arabinoside	Thiazides
Erythromycin esters	Thiourea
Fluorocytosine	Thioxanthenes
Methimazole	Tricyclic antidepressants
Methyltestosterone	Tolbutamide
Methylthiourea	Xenelamine
Naproxen	
Nicotinic acid	

[a] This list is not exhaustive. Consult other sources (see Suggested Further Reading). M, Mixed pattern, i.e. the whole range of biochemical parameters may be abnormal.

9.8 Hepatocellular agents

Although the main biochemical abnormality in chemically-induced hepatocellular injury is a high serum aminotransferase activity (Chapter 2), agents that primarily damage hepatocytes rarely do so without also causing some derangement of the cholestatic indices. The GGTP is the most sensitive of these indicators and can be quite markedly elevated. Serum ALP activities tend to be increased to a lesser extent and bilirubin concentrations may begin to rise after severe liver-cell damage has occurred. Of the drugs to which predominantly hepatocellular liver damage has been attributed (Table 9.4), paracetamol (acetaminophen) is perhaps the best example and has been extensively studied (Section 9.10). When taken in overdose, this drug causes hepatocellular necrosis and serum aminotransferase and GGTP activities 5 to 10 times the upper normal limit are often seen within 24 h but the ALP may be only moderately raised (two- to five-fold) and bilirubin concentrations are often normal. The serum bilirubin does not usually become grossly elevated until after about 36

TABLE 9.4. Examples of drugs that can cause a predominantly hepatocellular pattern of LFT abnormalities[a]

Acetohexamide (M)	Methyldopa
Allopurinol (M)	Niridazole
Antimonials	Novobiocin
Aprindin (M)	Oxyphenisatin
Carbutamide (M)	Papaverine
Chloramphenicol (M)	p-Aminosalicylic acid
Cincophen	Paracetamol
Clindamycin	Perhexiline maleate
Co-trimoxazole (M)	Phenylbutazone
Colchicine	Piperazine
Dantrolene	Probenicid
Phenytoin	Procainamide (M)
Ethionamide	Propylthiouracil
Gold (M)	Pyrazinamide
Hycanthone	Quinidine (M)
Hydralazine (M)	Rifampicin
Ibuprofen (M)	Salicylates
Indomethacin (M)	Sulphonamides (M)
Isoniazid	Tetracyclines (M)
MAO inhibitors	Thiosemicarbazone
Mepacrine	Tycrinafin
Metahexamide (M)	Valproate
Methotrexate	

[a] This list is not exhaustive. Consult other sources (see Suggested Further Reading). M, Mixed pattern, i.e. the whole range of biochemical parameters may be abnormal.

to 72 h, by which time aminotransferase activities of greater than 20 times normal may be recorded.

9.9 Anaesthetic agents

9.9.1 Halothane

Possibly because it has been so widely used, in recent years halothane has become the anaesthetic agent most frequently implicated as a cause of abnormal LFTs post-operatively. The exact frequency of *halothane hepatitis* is unknown, but severe (often fatal) hepatic damage reportedly occurs in about 1 in 35 000 anaesthetics and in about 1 in 3700 patients receiving multiple exposures. Less-severe clinical hepatitis probably occurs more often and minor (two- to four-fold) elevations in serum aminotransferases are common. The difficulties in precisely defining the frequency relate partly to the often transient nature of the less-severe abnormalities (which may be missed) and partly to the problem of distinguishing between a halothane-induced abnormality and the many other potential causes of post-operative elevations of serum aminotransferases. There is also the difficulty of documenting exposure, because the tubing of anaesthetic machines may retain residual amounts of halothane and patients given other anaesthetic agents using the same equipment may therefore receive small doses of halothane that could be significant in the present context.

The severe reaction to halothane is idiosyncratic [2]. Usually more than one exposure to the anaesthetic is required but abnormal LFTs have been documented after a single exposure. The biochemical abnormalities indicate hepatocellular damage, with elevated aminotransferases as the dominant feature, and tend to become progressively more severe with each subsequent exposure to halothane. In the full halothane hepatitis syndrome, other abnormal laboratory findings include eosinophilia (frequent) and, occasionally, one or more non-organ-specific autoantibodies (Chapter 6). Anti-LSP antibodies (Chapter 6) are found at high titre in about half of the patients during the acute phase. More specifically, a serum antibody that reacts with a rabbit liver antigen altered *in vivo* by halothane can be detected, but the techniques involved are fairly complicated and, so far, are available in only a very few specialized laboratories.

Because of the high mortality of halothane hepatitis, current recommendations are that patients who show a rise in serum aminotransferases post-operatively (whatever the suspected reason) should not be exposed to halothane again and that, as a general rule, multiple halothane anaesthesia should be avoided if possible.

9.9.2 Other agents

Chloroform is a predictable hepatotoxin and *methoxyflurane* will also cause liver damage but neither is any longer used widely. *Trichloroethylene (Trilene)* is potentially hepatotoxic but not usually at the concentrations used in anaesthesia (see also Section 9.19). *Enflurane* hepatitis is a well-recognized phenomenon but is much rarer than that caused by halothane. *Cyclopropane* has not been shown to cause liver injury.

9.10 Analgesics

9.10.1 Paracetamol (acetaminophen)

Paracetamol is currently the most common cause of death related to drug-induced liver damage in the UK, where the drug is used in overdose by individuals with suicidal intent. There is no evidence that this normally safe and effective drug causes any significant liver injury when taken alone at doses of less than 5 g, but above this level it is a predictable, indirect hepatotoxin (Section 9.3) and its toxicity is increased by inducing agents such as alcohol [3], phenobarbitone and phenytoin (Section 9.2.1).

Hepatic damage occurs at the time that the initial bolus of the overdose reaches the liver and is a consequence of massive depletion of glutathione, which is consumed during metabolism of the paracetamol. Serum aminotransferase activities rise sharply (two- to five-fold) within a few hours of ingestion and continue to increase, frequently to greater than 20 times the upper normal limit after three to five days. The serum GGTP and ALP activities follow the aminotransferases, but none of these enzymes (individually or in combination) is especially useful for prognosis in this situation. The serum bilirubin concentrations initially rise more slowly, with jaundice not usually beginning to appear until about 36 to 48 h after ingestion.

It is important to recognize that individuals who take an overdose of paracetamol may remain apparently well for many hours (or even two or three days) before they begin to develop symptoms of liver damage, for oral methionine or intravenous N-acetylcysteine as glutathione precursors are effective antidotes, *if given early*. N-acetylcysteine (Parvolcx) is the preferred antidote because it can be effective even when given up to 16 h after the overdose (Fig. 9.1), unlike oral methionine which must be administered within 12 h and tends to induce vomiting.

An accurate history of the amount of paracetamol taken is often difficult to obtain but knowledge of the amount of the drug ingested is not, in any event, a particularly useful prognostic index because the magnitude of the dose reaching the liver varies between individuals according to the rate of absorption. The plasma concentration of paracetamol and its clearance rate are more reliable indices. Patients with high plasma paracetamol concentrations (>1.0 mmol l^{-1} at 6 h and >0.2 mmol l^{-1} at 14 h after ingestion) will invariably suffer severe

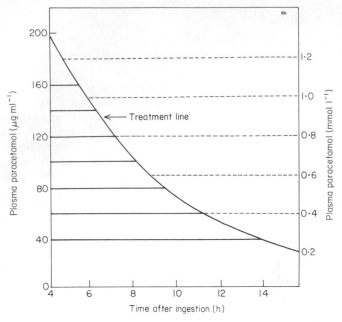

FIG 9.1. Plasma paracetamol (acetaminophen) concentrations following an overdose of the drug. If the concentration is above the "treatment line" at the times shown, severe liver damage is very likely and *N*-acetylcysteine must be administered immediately.

liver damage and *N*-acetylcysteine must be given immediately (Fig. 9.1).

The prothrombin time is also a very useful index in this situation. It rapidly becomes prolonged when liver damage occurs and is the first parameter to begin to return towards normal when the liver starts to recover its synthetic functions. Prothrombin ratios (INR) exceeding 5·0 are common but even lower ratios (INR > 2·2), particularly if accompanied by high (> 70 μmol l^{-1}) serum bilirubin concentrations, are a bad prognostic sign. Such patients can be expected to develop fulminant hepatic failure, which has a high mortality rate. *It cannot be emphasized too strongly that early referral of such patients to a centre with specialist intensive-care facilities is essential.* Experience in our Unit has shown that prognosis is especially poor when the prothrombin time is > 100 s and the blood pH is < 7·3 on admission and measures to prevent patients reaching this stage must be instituted early.

Measurements of plasma ammonia, mercaptans and other metabolites are largely of academic interest, but the plasma urea and creatinine should be monitored to warn of impending renal failure, which is a complication as common in this situation as in acute liver failure due to other causes (Chapter 3).

9.10.2   Other analgesics

Like paracetamol, other analgesics do not cause liver damage when taken in normal therapeutic doses but problems can arise when these agents are taken in larger amounts [4]. Thus, *aspirin* in doses exceeding $2\,g\,day^{-1}$ tends to be a predictable hepatotoxin. Damage is predominantly hepatocellular, with raised serum aminotransferases and normal or only mildly elevated serum bilirubin concentrations or ALP activities, and may occur in 20% or more of patients at this dose level. Aspirin has also been implicated as a cause of chronic hepatitis, with features virtually indistinguishable from autoimmune chronic active hepatitis (see Chapter 6).

Of the other drugs in this group, only *dextropropoxyphene* has been reported (occasionally) as causing liver damage (either cholestatic or hepatocellular) at higher therapeutic doses but most analgesics are capable of causing some hepatic injury when taken in overdose.

9.11   Anti-convulsants

Phenytoin (*diphenylhydantoin, dilantin*) and *sodium valproate* (n-dipropyl-acetic acid) are the two most widely used drugs in this category. Both can be hepatotoxic. About 20% of patients taking phenytoin show persistent mild elevations of serum aminotransferases and/or ALP, but occasionally patients (mainly adult females) can develop a severe hepatitic illness with very high aminotransferase and ALP activities and with clinical symptoms suggesting a hypersensitivity reaction, which often progesses to fulminant hepatic failure. Sodium valproate seems to be somewhat less toxic. About 10% of patients receiving the drug reportedly show mild elevations in serum aminotransferases. Very occasionally, however, a severe hypersensitivity type of acute hepatitis with markedly raised aminotransferases (similar to that seen with phenytoin) can develop (with often fatal consequences), particularly in children and in those with underlying metabolic disorders, where hyperammonaemia may be an additional sign of hepatotoxicity. *Carbamazepine* has been reported occasionally to cause cholestatic jaundice and agranulocytosis, leucopenia and thrombocytopenia.

9.12   Anti-inflammatory drugs

Paracetamol and salicylates have been discussed above (Section 9.10) and steroidal agents are considered below (Section 9.16). Of the other commonly used anti-inflammatory drugs, many seem to be hepatotoxic to at least some extent. *Dantrolene, ibuprofen, indomethacin, naproxen, phenylbutazone* and its derivatives, *penicillamine* and even *gold* have all been reported to cause cholestasis with variable degrees of hepatocellular injury and the toxicity of *benoxyprophen* in the elderly is now well recognized. Phenylbutazone and oxyphenylbutazone in therapeutic doses can cause a hepatitic illness the clinical symptoms of which suggest a hypersensitivity reaction and the former has been suspected as a cause of chronic active hepatitis. In overdose, phenylbutazone can produce acute hepatic necrosis. *Sulindac* can also, reportedly, cause a cholestatic hepatitis (with or without jaundice) with fever and rashes or other skin reactions suggestive of hypersensitivity.

Considering how extensively these drugs are used, however, overt liver damage is quite rare. Nevertheless, a high proportion of patients receiving these and other anti-inflammatory agents at normal doses show persistent mild abnormalities of LFTs suggestive of some degree of chronic cholestasis.

The biochemical abnormalities mainly comprise only slight elevations in ALP and GGTP. Serum aminotransferase activities and bilirubin concentrations are usually normal but activities of another (less commonly used) serum marker of hepatocellular damage, *ornithine carbamoyl transferase*, have been found to be elevated in up to 20% of rheumatoid patients on gold or phenylbutazone therapy. It might be expected that, in the rheumatic diseases, the ALP would be of bone origin but, paradoxically, this seems not to be the case. In our experience [5], the total ALP activity in almost 90% of rheumatoid arthritis patients is attributable wholly or mainly to the liver iso-enzyme, even in patients with normal ALP activities.

Serum autoantibody measurements are of little value in investigating suspected hepatotoxicity of anti-inflammatory agents, because many of the disorders in which these drugs are used are themselves associated with a high frequency of autoantibodies.

9.13 Antimicrobial agents

9.13.1 Antibiotics

The hepatotoxic potential of the *tetracyclines* is well known and has been extensively studied. They are predictable hepatotoxins but overt liver damage is rarely seen at doses of less than $2\,g\,day^{-1}$. At higher doses (e.g. when given intravenously), tetracyclines can give rise to an illness that, clinically and biochemically, is very similar to acute viral hepatitis and which is often associated with progressive renal failure and pancreatitis. In addition to increases in the serum aminotransferases and the cholestatic indices, the laboratory findings usually include elevated blood urea concentrations and serum amylase activities, a metabolic acidosis, hypoglycaemia and a leucocytosis. Liver biopsies show excessive fat deposition similar to that seen in acute fatty liver of pregnancy. It should be noted that, since tetracyclines are normally eliminated via the kidney, subjects with pre-existing renal disease may suffer liver damage even at relatively low doses.

Erythromycin is not in itself hepatotoxic but its esters, *erythromycin estolate* and *ethylsuccinate* and *triacetyloleandomycin* (which are no longer widely used), have all been implicated as occasional causes of liver damage. The laboratory picture is usually that of a cholestatic hepatitis, with only moderate (<10-fold) elevations in serum aminotransferases, and is often associated with an eosinophilia. The latter, together with an urticarial rash which is a common presenting symptom, suggests that toxicity is related to hypersensitivity.

The *sulphonamides* (including *sulphasalazine*) are all potentially hepatotoxic and can give rise to hepatitic illnesses with laboratory findings and clinical features of hypersensitivity that are similar to those produced by the *erythromycin esters*. The level of toxicity of the *sulphonamides* is generally low but can be enhanced by inducing agents (Section 9.2.1) taken concurrently.

Like the sulphonamides, *nitrofurantoin* has occasionally been associated with hepatitic illness with features of hypersensitivity [6] and it has been suggested that this drug may also cause chronic active hepatitis. In contrast, the "hepatotoxicity" of *novobiocin*, usually manifested by elevated serum bilirubin concentrations, is thought to be due to interference with bilirubin transport.

The severe hypersensitivity reactions commonly seen with *penicillin* itself are only very rarely associated with hepatic damage but other penicillins, such as *carbenicillin*, *oxacillin* and *phenoxymethyl penicillin*, reportedly cause parenchymal liver injury (with or without cholestasis) occasionally when given in large doses intravenously. *Co-trimoxazole* (*Septrin*) often causes mild elevations in ALP and GGTP, but instances of hyperbilirubinaemia and severe liver damage seem to be very rare.

9.13.2 Antituberculous drugs

p-Aminosalicylic acid (PAS) is a drug to which up to 15% of patients become sensitized and up to 25% of these develop hepatic damage. Patients exhibit the usual symptoms of generalized hypersensitivity (fever, rashes, arthralgia) and eosinophilia is common. In those with liver damage, the laboratory tests indicate hepatocellular injury (often quite severe and sometimes fatal), with high activities of serum aminotransferases and ALP. *Rifampicin* and *isoniazid* are both hepatotoxic. The former is an inducing agent (Section 9.2.1) and considerably enhances the toxicity of isoniazid when the two drugs are used together. This synergistic action is also seen with PAS but to a lesser extent because PAS is an inhibitor of MFOS enzymes (Section 9.2) and reportedly actually reduces the toxic effects of both rifampicin and isoniazid. When these drugs are taken separately, up to 4% of patients receiving rifampicin and about 1% of those taking isoniazid develop severe liver damage with features of acute viral hepatitis.

Rifampicin competes with bilirubin for transport across the liver cell and conjugated or unconjugated hyperbilirubinaemia can often occur as the sole biochemical abnormality but, in cases of severe hepatotoxicity, will normally be accompanied by high serum aminotransferase activities. With isoniazid, the laboratory findings are similar to those seen in PAS-induced liver damage, i.e. serum aminotransferases, ALP and GGTP tending to be elevated to a greater extent than is the serum bilirubin.

Many patients (up to 20%) taking rifampicin and/or isoniazid develop mild to moderate abnormalities of one or more biochemical indices of liver injury which resolve spontaneously despite continuation of the drugs. However, there is evidence to suggest that liver damage may continue in some of these patients even after their LFTs return towards normality. Those in whom the biochemical abnormalities persist may develop features of chronic active hepatitis if the drug is not discontinued.

Pyrazinamide is so hepatotoxic that it is no longer used. *Ethionamide* can cause liver damage similar to that seen with *isoniazid* but reportedly much less frequently. *Cycloserine, ethambutol* and *streptomycin* seem not to be hepatotoxic.

9.13.3   Antihelminthics and other antimicrobials

The organic antimonials and chlorinated hydrocarbons, used as antihelminthics, have long been known to cause liver damage. The antischistosomal drugs *hycanthone* and *niridazole* have been found to produce hepatocellular necrosis, as has *piperazine*. *Thiobendazole* has been implicated as the causative agent in a few cases of intrahepatic cholestasis with features resembling those of primary biliary cirrhosis. Other drugs, such as the *sulphones* used in the treatment of leprosy, *clindamycin*, and the antifungal agent *griseofulvin*, have only occasionally been found to cause liver damage but another antifungal agent, *ketoconazole*, has been reported to cause hepatitis, particularly when given for longer periods (>two weeks) and will exacerbate pre-existing liver disease.

Among the anti-viral agents, information on hepatotoxicity is scanty but there are reports that *idoxyuridine, xenelamine* and *cytosine arabinoside* sometimes produce cholestasis. Most of the drugs used in the treatment of amoebiasis and other protozoan infections seem not to be overtly hepatotoxic. However, the hepatotoxicity of the antimalarial agent, *amodiaquin* (*4-aminoquinoline*), is well recognized and fatalities following amodiaquin-induced fulminant hepatitis have been reported [7]. Another antimalarial drug, *pyrimethamine*, may induce hepatotoxicity when taken concurrently with the benzodiazepine *lorazepam*. Short-term use of pyrimethamine in patients with liver diseases may not carry an increased risk but long-term prophylactic use is contraindicated in such patients, as it can cause bone-marrow depression and will exacerbate folate deficiency.

9.14 Antineoplastic drugs

Several of the drugs used in cancer chemotherapy are hepatotoxic. In view of the doubtful hepatotoxicity of *azathioprine* (Section 9.17), it is perhaps surprising that there have been several reports implicating its metabolite, *6-mercaptopurine*, as a cause of both severe cholestasis and of hepatocellular necrosis. This seems to be particularly the case when 6-mercaptopurine is given in conjunction with *adriamycin* (*doxorubicin*), although the latter appears not to be directly hepatotoxic itself. Other drugs in this category that are said to cause liver damage include *6-chloropurine*, *thioguanine*, *azaserine*, *bleomycin*, *mitomycin*, *puromycin C*, *5-fluorouracil*, *chlorambucil*, *cyclophosphamide* and *methotrexate* (Section 9.16), while others such as *actinomycin D*, *cycloheximide* and *daunorubicin* are rarely (if ever) hepatotoxic.

9.15 Cardiovascular drugs

Up to 35% of patients taking *methyldopa* reportedly show mildly abnormal LFTs. Severe liver damage is relatively uncommon but is widely recognized. "*Methyldopa hepatitis*" often has an acute onset very closely resembling acute viral hepatitis, both clinically and biochemically, with serum aminotransferase activities frequently exceeding 20 times the upper normal limit. In some patients, the onset is more insidious but, whatever the pattern of presentation, continued use of the drug can lead to a condition that is virtually indistinguishable from autoimmune chronic active hepatitis (Chapter 6) with LE cell phenomena, hyperglobulinaemia, non-organ-specific autoantibodies and anti-LSP antibodies (Chapter 6). Biochemically, the findings are usually typical of predominantly hepatocellular injury, but occasionally patients may present a more cholestatic picture.

Liver damage due to another widely used antihypertensive drug, *hydralazine*, seems to be very rare but has been documented. Patients taking this drug may show mild abnormalities of LFTs suggesting either cholestatic or hepatocellular disease, but occasionally the abnormalities can be quite marked and the term *hydralazine "pseudo-lupus"* has been used to describe this syndrome.

Among the antiarrhythmia agents, *quinidine* hypersensitivity is now well recognized. This drug can cause haemolytic anaemia as well as (less commonly) hepatic damage. Thus patients may develop unconjugated and/or conjugated hyperbilirubinaemia. Minor increases in serum aminotransferase and ALP activities are relatively common, but eosinophilia appears not to be a feature of quinidine toxicity. *Procainamide* and *aprindine* seem to be very rarely hepatotoxic but *ajmaline* (derived from the plant *Rauwolfia serpentina*), like quinidine, has been implicated more often as a cause of liver injury. The reported biochemical abnormalities associated with ajmaline hepatotoxicity range from the purely cholestatic to predominantly hepatocellular and it has been said that the syndrome can mimic primary biliary cirrhosis.

Amiodarone is known to be hepatotoxic. Transient elevations of the liver enzymes are not uncommon but usually respond to reduction in dose. However, very occasionally severe liver damage may occur and may progress to cirrhosis despite withdrawal of the drug. Current recommendations are that LFTs should be performed before commencing treatment and should be monitored at regular intervals thereafter. A peripheral neuropathy, tremor and ataxia are additional side-effects and, in patients with abnormal LFTs, the overall picture may be confused with that of alcoholic liver disease.

A number of other drugs currently used for treatment of cardiovascular disease are hepatotoxic. The anticoagulant *phenindione* is a well-documented (but fairly rare) cause of liver damage (with a biochemical picture of cholestatic hepatitis), and fatalities have been reported, but other anticoagulants have been only very infrequently implicated. The *thiazide* diuretics also very occasionally cause hepatic injury but their wide use in patients with pre-existing liver disease is an indication of their generally low hepatotoxicity. However, another diuretic, *ticrynafin*, has been found to produce hepatic damage with up to 40-fold elevations in serum aminotransferases (with or without abnormalities in the cholestatic indices) and has now been withdrawn in some countries.

Perhexiline maleate, used to treat angina pectoris, produces mild elevations of serum aminotransferases in up to 50% of patients but overt liver damage (resembling alcoholic hepatitis and leading to cirrhosis) seems to occur only in a small proportion of these.

The antihyperlipidaemic agents almost all show some degree of hepatotoxicity. *Clofibrate* is associated with a low incidence of mild elevations in serum aminotransferases, which is thought to be of muscle origin because of concomitant increases in creatine kinase, but there are reports of occasional hepatocellular injury and of "granulomatous hepatitis" (Chapter 12). *Nicotinic acid* reportedly causes abnormal liver function tests in up to 50% of patients on long-term treatment and overt liver damage with markedly raised serum bilirubin and aminotransferases in about 5%.

9.16 Endocrinological agents

Of all the drugs that cause cholestasis, probably the most frequently encountered are the C-17 alkylated steroids and related compounds that have an unsaturated phenolic A ring. Almost the entire range of anabolic, progestational and oestrogenic agents has been implicated, but the mechanisms are poorly understood. *Testosterone* (which has no substituent at C-17) does not induce cholestasis but *methyltestosterone* (which differs only by having a methyl group at C-17) does. On the other hand, *oestradiol* (which does not have a C-17 substituent) appears to interfere with bilirubin transport. This seems to be related to the highly unsaturated state of the phenolic A ring of *oestradiol*.

Women taking oral contraceptives containing C-17 *ethinyloestrogen* and *progesterone* derivatives can sometimes show mild (but apparently benign) elevations in serum bilirubin concentrations, but the possibility that this may be due to undiagnosed *Gilbert's syndrome* must be considered (see Chapter 2). More pronounced elevations (30–50 μmol l^{-1}) accompanied by increased ALP activities are usually associated with symptoms of hepatobiliary disease. In these cases, there are often also mild elevations (200–300 IU l^{-1}) in the serum aminotransferases but occasionally activities may exceed 1000 IU l^{-1}. Usually these abnormalities slowly resolve when the drug is stopped. If they persist after withdrawing the drug, it is likely that the abnormalities are due to a more serious underlying disorder, such as Budd–Chiari syndrome (from hepatic venous occlusion due to the thrombogenic effects of oestrogenic components), a benign hepatic tumour (adenoma) or some other complication.

Nevertheless, considering how many millions of women have been taking oral contraceptives over the past 25 years, the frequency of such complications is very low indeed. This is not the case with the *C-17 substituted androgenic-anabolic steroids*, all of which produce cholestasis in a dose-related manner and many of which lead to development of hepatocellular carcinoma and other serious conditions, e.g. peliosis hepatis, when used for prolonged periods.

Among the drugs used for treating endocrine disorders, the oral hypoglycaemic agents are probably the most hepatotoxic. Asymptomatic, transient elevations in ALP and/or serum bilirubin are quite often seen in patients taking these drugs. Actual hepatic damage reportedly occurs in about 1% of patients receiving *chlorpropamide, carbutamide, metaheximide* or *acetoheximide*. *Tolbutamide* has been less often implicated but, like chlorpropamide, it appears to produce a "pure" cholestasis (i.e. with only mild elevations in the serum markers of hepatocellular injury) and this has been said to progress to a syndrome resembling primary biliary cirrhosis. Toxicity due to carbutamide and the heximides tends to be associated with abnormalities in the whole range of biochemical LFTs. Eosinophilia is common and the clinical symptoms suggest hypersensitivity.

The antithyroid drugs seem to be much less hepatotoxic than the oral hypoglycaemic agents but *thiouracil, methylthiouracil, methimazole* and *carbimazole* have all been reported to cause cholestasis (with or without elevations in serum aminotransferases), while *propylthiouracil* can produce hepatocellular necrosis with biochemical and histological features of chronic active hepatitis. The hepatotoxic manifestations of the *thiourea* derivatives are often accompanied by eosinophilia, neutropenia and clinical signs of hypersensitivity.

9.17 Immunosuppressive drugs

The hepatotoxicity of *methotrexate*, widely used in the treatment of severe psoriasis, is well recognized and seems to be exacerbated by concomitant alcohol consumption or complicating factors such as obesity or diabetes. Increased serum aminotransferase and ALP activities are common but even patients with normal LFTs can develop hepatic steatosis and fibrosis that may progress to cirrhosis. For this reason, it is becoming the practice to assess hepatic function by liver biopsy at the start of treatment and periodically thereafter. The histological picture in methotrexate-induced liver damage together with a cholestatic pattern of biochemical liver function tests can be confused with alcoholic liver disease.

Azathioprine is widely employed in the treatment of liver disease and appears to be relatively safe at the dosages (1 or $2\,\text{mg}\,\text{kg}^{-1}$) used, but there is quite good evidence that it is hepatotoxic at higher doses. In our experience, patients with pre-existing liver disease treated with azathioprine for many years develop at most only mild elevations in serum bilirubin, ALP or GGTP that can be attributed to the drug. Nevertheless, there have been reports of more severe liver damage which may be due to an idiosyncratic reaction to azathioprine. In addition, the drug does cause myelosuppression in some patients even at low doses and it is recommended that full blood counts be performed at regular intervals.

Cyclosporin is becoming more commonly used in patients with liver disease and is now the drug of choice in recipients of liver grafts. This drug is hepatotoxic to some extent but its nephrotoxicity is a more important problem and serum creatinine should, therefore, be monitored regularly in patients receiving cyclosporin.

Unlike the steroidal agents discussed above (Section 9.16), the corticosteroids such as *prednisolone* which are so widely used in the treatment of autoimmune and other hyperallergic conditions seem not to be hepatotoxic.

9.18 Psychotropic drugs

Psychotropic drugs are well-known hepatotoxins. The *phenothiazines, benzodiazepines* and *tricyclic anti-depressants* tend to be cholestatic agents while *monoamine oxidase inhibitors* are more likely to produce hepatocellular damage.

Chlorpromazine jaundice is a particularly well-recognized complication and up to 2% of patients taking this drug are likely to develop the syndrome. Many more show mild elevations in serum bilirubin, usually with concomitant increases in ALP and/or GGTP. In the full syndrome, bilirubin concentrations can reach $250 \mu mol\, l^{-1}$ and ALP is generally increased at least five-fold but serum aminotransferase activities are usually only moderately elevated (two- to five-fold). The clinical features of jaundice and pruritis, together with the occasional finding of antimitochondrial antibodies (Chapter 6) in the serum, can lead to confusion with primary biliary cirrhosis.

The lower reported frequency of liver damage with other phenothiazines probably reflects their less-common use. The *benzodiazepines* can also cause a cholestatic hepatitis, sometimes accompanied by eosinophilia and clinical symptoms of a viral infection, as can the *tricyclic antidepressants*. However, considering the widespread use of both these classes of drugs, reports of such complications are quite rare.

All of the *monoamine oxidase inhibitors* are hepatotoxic but the *hydrazine* derivatives, such as *iproniazid*, are the best documented. Up to 2% of patients receiving these drugs may develop a severe acute hepatitis (often fatal), with markedly raised (>10-fold) serum aminotransferases, but many more show milder elevations in these enzymes and/or ALP and GGTP. Those taking *iproniazid* may develop the "pseudo-lupus" syndrome with antimitochondrial antibodies (Chapter 6).

9. DRUGS AND OTHER CHEMICAL HEPATOTOXINS

9.19 Occupational, environmental and other agents

The list of potential hepatotoxins with which we come into contact in our daily lives is far too long to reproduce here and only a few examples are given to illustrate the range of these compounds.

Obvious candidates are the halogenated hydrocarbons so widely encountered in industry and the home, most of which can cause varying degrees of cholestasis and/or hepatocellular injury in a predictable manner. This category includes the normally safe anaesthetic agent *trichloroethylene* (*Trilene*), which is also used as a solvent in adhesives and has been known to cause liver damage in young people indulging in the practice of "glue-sniffing", and *carbon tetrachloride*, accidental poisoning with which is still occasionally reported.

Some pesticides, such as *chlordecone*, and many compounds used in the paint and plastics industries cause hepatic injury in various ways. Classical examples of the latter are *diaminodiphenylmethane*, accidental ingestion of which led to an epidemic of jaundice at Epping in England, and *vinyl chloride* (which is carcinogenic).

In the plant world, there are numerous compounds that are hepatotoxic in man. These range from the *Senecio* and *Heliotropium alkaloids* (which cause veno-occlusive disease) to the mushroom toxins (of which that produced by the "black cap" mushroom, *Amanita phalloides*, is perhaps the most frequent cause of mushroom poisoning) and to substances such as *aflatoxin*. The latter is produced by a fungus that commonly grows on ground-nuts stored under damp conditions. It is a potent carcinogen and, at higher doses, can be directly hepatotoxic.

A number of substances used in medical practice have also been found to cause liver injury. Most of these, such as the radiological contrast agent *Thorotrast* (which caused cirrhosis and hepatic tumours) and *tannic acid* (a constituent of barium enema preparations which caused hepatocellular necrosis), are now obsolete. However, a few others are still in use, albeit to a limited extent. Examples include the cholecystographic agent *bunamiodyl* (which interferes with bilirubin transport and can cause a mild unconjugated hyperbilirubinaemia) and *oxyphenisatin*, a laxative which has largely been withdrawn from general use but is still included as a component of some enemas used preparatory to bowel examinations. This latter drug was found to produce, particularly in women, a syndrome in which the biochemical, histological, immunological and clinical features were virtually indistinguishable from autoimmune chronic active hepatitis (even progressing to cirrhosis in some cases) but which slowly resolved when the drug was discontinued.

203

References

1. Coon MJ and Koop DR. Arch Toxicol 1987; 60: 16.
2. Neuberger J and Kenna JG. Clin Sci 1987; 72: 263.
3. Maddrey WC. J Clin Gastroenterol 1987; 9: 180.
4. Cersosimo RJ and Matthews SJ. Drug Intell Clin Pharmacol 1987; 21: 62.
5. Fernandes L et al. Ann Rheum Dis 1979; 38: 501.
6. Stricker BHC. Hepatology 1988; 8: 599.
7. Bernuau J et al. J Hepatol 1988; 6: 109.

Suggested further reading

Blei AT. Pharmacokinetic-hemodynamic interactions in cirrhosis. Semin Liver Dis 6: 299–308.

Gibson GG and Skett P. Principles of Biochemical Toxicology. London: Chapman & Hall, 1986.

Kenna JG, Neuberger J and Williams R. Evidence for expression in human liver of halothane-induced neoantigens recognized by antibodies in sera from patients with halothane hepatitis. Hepatology 1988; 8: 1635–1641.

Ludwig J and Axelsen R. Drug effects on the liver: an updated tabular compilation of drugs and drug-related hepatic diseases. Dig Disease Sci 1983; 28: 651–666.

Nerbert DW and Gonzalez FJ. P450 genes: structure evolution and regulation. Ann Rev Biochem 1987; 56: 945–993.

Neuberger J and Kenna JG. Halothane hepatitis: a model of immune mediated drug hepatotoxicity. Clin Sci 1987; 72: 263–270.

Secor JW and Schenker S. Drug metabolism in patients with liver disease. Adv Intern Med 1987; 32: 379–405.

Stricker BHC and Spoelstra P. Drug-induced hepatic injury. In: Drug-Induced Disorders, Vol. 1 (Dukes MNG, Ed). Amsterdam: Elsevier, 1985.

Timbrell JA. Principles of Biochemical Toxicology. London: Taylor & Francis, 1985.

Weber WW and Hein DW. N-acetylation pharmacogenetics. Pharmacol Revs 1985; 37: 25–79.

Zimmerman HJ. Hepatotoxicity: The Adverse Effects of Drugs and Other Chemicals on the Liver. New York: Appleton-Century-Crofts, 1978.

10

Alcohol and liver disease

10.1   Introduction

Where alcohol in relation to liver disease is concerned, the clinician is usually faced with one of three problems. (i) Does a patient with a history of heavy alcohol consumption have underlying liver disease? (ii) In a patient who is known to be a heavy drinker and has evidence of liver damage, is the damage in fact due to the alcohol? [1, 2]. (iii) Could undisclosed heavy alcohol consumption be the cause of idiopathic liver disease in a professed abstainer? In each instance, the problem is compounded by the notorious difficulty of accurately documenting alcohol consumption and by the wide variability between individuals in their susceptibility to alcoholic liver damage. Not infrequently, patients with alcoholic liver disease have no symptoms of liver damage and this may be revealed only serendipitously (e.g. on routine health screening). On the other hand, in the patient with evidence of liver disease who freely admits to "having a few drinks occasionally", it may be tempting to interpret what may be an honest and accurate admission as an indication of alcohol abuse and to look no further for the cause of the liver damage.

There is at present no test or combination of tests that unequivocally differentiates between alcohol-induced and other forms of liver disease. Random blood or urine alcohol analysis can be helpful in documenting alcohol ingestion when this is denied by the patient, but gives no information about the nature or severity of any underlying liver damage. Other laboratory findings will depend upon the nature of the alcohol-induced liver injury and their interpretation will be influenced by whether the patient presents with an acute illness or, as is more often the case, with somewhat vague signs or symptoms that do not immediately suggest alcohol as a cause. However, there are several biochemical and other laboratory abnormalities that tend to be associated with alcohol-induced liver disease and which together can form a pattern that at least raises the suspicion of an alcoholic aetiology (see Section 10.6).

10.2 Factors contributing to alcoholic liver injury

The form in which alcohol is consumed (beer, wine, spirits, etc.) is largely irrelevant. Rather, it is the total amount of alcohol ingested together with the duration of drinking and individual susceptibility that determine whether (and to what degree) the liver will be damaged. Episodic bouts of heavy drinking (> 300 g ethanol/day) may sometimes lead to acute alcoholic hepatitis (see below), but, if interspersed by periods of abstinence, are unlikely to result in chronic liver disease which is more usually the consequence of the regular daily consumption of somewhat lesser amounts of alcohol over prolonged periods. There is no evidence that a regular intake of $10-15$ g day^{-1} leads to any significant liver damage but the risk of developing cirrhosis increases about five-fold at 50 g day^{-1} [3] and is more than 25-fold when the daily

TABLE 10.1. The approximate ethanol content of common alcoholic beverages

		Ethanol content (g)
Beer	per pint (Imp.)	25
Table wines	per glass (125 ml)	15
	per bottle (75 cl)	90
Fortified wines	per glass (75 ml)	15
(sherry, port, etc.)	per bottle (75 cl)	150
Spirits	per fl. oz. (28 ml)	11
(whisky, gin, etc.)	per bottle (75 cl)	280
Liqueurs	per glass (60 ml)	16
	per bottle (75 cl)	200

intake exceeds 100 g (equivalent to about one-third of a bottle of spirits; see Table 10.1).

Women seem to be more susceptible than men to alcohol-related liver damage, even when differences in body weight are taken into account, and tend to develop cirrhosis at lower daily alcohol intakes over shorter periods [4]. This may be due partly to differences in body composition (e.g. higher body fat/weight ratio than in men) and partly to hormonal differences. In addition, the fact that some individuals can consume fairly large amounts of alcohol over many years without any significant liver injury while others develop cirrhosis after much shorter periods on lower alcohol intakes is taken to indicate that genetic factors may be involved. This is supported by several reports of apparent associations between the development of alcohol-induced liver injury and certain histocompatibility (HLA) antigens, but these markers differ between the various populations studied [5, 6]. Of interest is a reported association with HLA B8 [7, 8], which is a marker that is common in several autoimmune disorders. This, together with the finding of various auto-antibodies in a proportion of patients (Section 10.6.4), suggests that immunological mechanisms may underlie the development of cirrhosis in some cases. Other genetic factors that might determine susceptibility relate to differences between individuals in isoenzymes of the alcohol and/or aldehyde dehydrogenases involved in the metabolism of ethanol.

10.3   Metabolism of alcohol

Approximately 90% of any ethanol ingested is metabolized by the liver. The rate-limiting step is the conversion of alcohol to acetaldehyde. This reaction can be catalysed by a number of enzymes, including components of the mixed-function oxidase system (MFOS, Chapter 9), but alcohol dehydrogenase (ADH) is quantitatively the most important. The acetaldehyde produced is then converted to acetate by aldehyde dehydrogenase (ALDH). NADH is generated in each of these two reactions and its increased availability (together with other metabolic effects of ethanol) favours production of lipids, ketones, lactate and porphyrins. This leads to fat deposition in hepatocytes, as well as hyperlipidaemia, ketosis, lacticacidaemia and, in some cases, porphyria (Chapter 11).

10.4   The spectrum of alcoholic liver damage

There are three principal histological categories of alcohol-induced liver injury: *fatty change*, *alcoholic hepatitis* and *fibrosis/cirrhosis* (Fig. 10.1). Each may be found alone or in combination with one or both of the other two and the clinical and laboratory findings, as well as prognosis, will depend on the existence (or co-existence) of these features.

It is not uncommon for normal or near-normal liver architecture to be found in liver biopsies from individuals who consume excessive amounts of alcohol (even when there is clinical evidence of hepatomegaly) but, as a consequence of the metabolic events outlined above, the majority of heavy drinkers will have some fat deposited in their livers. *Fatty liver* is the most benign of the alcohol-induced changes and is often reversible by avoiding alcohol, but it is very variable in severity. In its more severe forms, the fatty change can be accompanied by fibrous-tissue deposition (possibly leading to cirrhosis [9]) while, occasionally, large fat vacuoles may rupture hepatocytes and the ensuing inflammatory reaction can lead to development of lipogranulomata.

Alcoholic hepatitis is a more serious condition. It may present acutely, e.g. after a bout of particularly heavy drinking, or it may be insidious. The histological features include foci of (usually centrilobular) necrosis with a leucocytic infiltration (usually polymorphs) and cytoplasmic inclusions of a granular material, *Mallory's hyaline*.

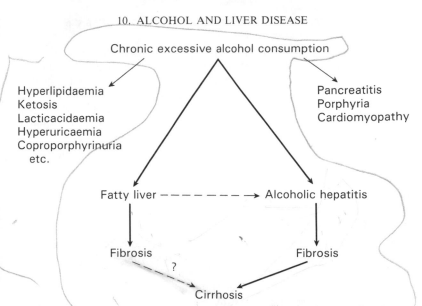

FIGURE 10.1. Stages in the development of alcoholic liver disease.

The latter is not, however, pathognomonic of alcoholic liver injury, since it is found in cirrhosis of other aetiologies (e.g. primary biliary cirrhosis). Alcoholic hepatitis will often resolve upon cessation of drinking but it can persist in some individuals who refrain from further alcohol intake and it predisposes to cirrhosis more frequently and more rapidly than does fatty liver alone. The combination of alcoholic hepatitis and cirrhosis (so-called "active" cirrhosis) can often present a histological picture very similar to that of chronic active hepatitis due to other causes [10].

Although the development of cirrhosis is an irreversible step, cessation of drinking may lead to an improvement in liver function. This is presumably due to diminution of "active", alcohol-induced liver damage and in such individuals the liver disease enters a quiescent phase ("inactive" cirrhosis) which may progress only very slowly over many years of continued abstinence.

10.5 Mechanisms of alcohol-induced liver injury

The precise mechanisms that lead to the various forms of alcohol-induced liver damage are poorly understood. As noted above, the accumulation of fat in hepatocytes is a relatively benign feature that probably does not cause significant hepatocellular injury on its own, except when the fat deposition is really excessive. It is possible that alcohol itself might directly damage hepatocytes but its main metabolite, acetaldehyde, is a more likely candidate for induction of such chemically-mediated tissue injury. Acetaldehyde is a highly reactive and toxic compound that inhibits cellular respiration and may be involved in the generation of toxic free radicals [11] that can cause peroxidation of membrane lipids, leading to loss of the functional integrity of cell membranes. It has been suggested that increased cellular concentrations of acetaldehyde might occur in some individuals as a result of genetic differences in the activities of the two principal enzymes (ADH and ALDH, see above) involved in alcohol metabolism, leading to overproduction of acetaldehyde or its slower conversion to acetate.

The inflammatory reaction in alcoholic hepatitis can arise as a response to cell death (induced perhaps by alcohol or acetaldehyde), but it is difficult to explain why it persists in some subjects even after cessation of drinking. This has raised the question of whether immunological mechanisms might be involved in certain susceptible individuals. Several studies have demonstrated that lymphocytes from patients with alcoholic hepatitis react against both normal and abnormal liver-cell components *in vitro*, and that such patients have circulating antibodies against "alcohol-altered" hepatocytes [12]. There is now also considerable evidence that acetaldehyde can bind covalently to hepatic macromolecules to form *neo*antigens, some of which may be expressed on hepatocellular surfaces, and that alcoholic patients have circulating antibodies that react with these adducts [13]. Concomitant autoimmune reactions triggered by these anti-adduct responses might account for the persistence of liver damage in some individuals even after they have stopped drinking.

A third hypothesis invokes environmental factors. It has been suggested that chronic alcohol consumption in some way makes the liver more susceptible to injury by microbial or chemical agents, but supporting evidence for such a mechanism has been slow to materialize.

10.6 Investigation of alcoholic liver disease

10.6.1 General considerations

The overlapping features and broad spectrum of alcohol-induced liver injury, together with the wide individual variability in response to excessive alcohol intake, makes the laboratory diagnosis of alcoholic liver disease exceedingly difficult and the presence and severity of tissue damage can really only be properly assessed by liver biopsy. This is not to say that there is little point in carrying out laboratory tests on a patient with suspected alcoholic liver disease, but the plan of investigation and, in particular, the interpretation of the results will depend upon which of the three questions posed in the Introduction to this chapter is being addressed.

In the patient with a history of excessive alcohol intake, the most useful investigations for underlying liver disease are probably the biochemical liver function tests (LFTs), the haematological parameters and the serum IgA (see below and Table 10.2). These are also probably the most useful investigations for excluding secret alcohol abuse as a cause of idiopathic liver disease in a patient who denies excessive alcohol consumption. In the patient who admits to heavy drinking, alcohol-related laboratory abnormalities may mask

TABLE 10.2. Laboratory findings that are suggestive of alcoholic liver disease[a]

Biochemistry	
GGTP	Increased out of proportion to other biochemical liver function tests
AST : ALT ratio	$> 2 : 1$
Serum cholesterol	Increased with or without increases in other classes of lipids
Haematology	
ESR	Raised
MCV	Increased
Macrocytosis	Present (often marked)
Plasma B_{12} and folate	Either or both decreased
Immunology	
Serum IgA	Increased (IgG may also be slightly increased but IgM is usually normal)
Urinalysis	
Coproporphyrins	Increased

[a] None of these abnormalities is specific for alcohol abuse but a combination of four or more spread between at least two of the above categories should raise the suspicion of alcoholic liver disease.

underlying liver disease of some other aetiology and in such individuals further investigations should be carried out to exclude other causes of any abnormalities detected (see Section 10.7). Whatever the reason for investigation, it is important to bear in mind that normal laboratory results do not automatically exclude alcohol-induced changes in the liver, especially fatty liver or inactive cirrhosis.

10.6.2   Biochemistry

10.6.2.1   Standard liver function tests

In *alcoholic hepatitis*, the biochemical LFTs are almost always deranged. Typically, the pattern of abnormalities indicates cholestasis, with moderately increased serum alkaline phosphatase (ALP) activities (up to five-fold) and bilirubin concentrations ($20-50\,\mu\text{mol}\,l^{-1}$), but either or both may be grossly elevated in patients with severe liver damage. The serum aspartate aminotransferase (AST) activity is characteristically moderately increased (usually $< 100\,\text{IU}\,l^{-1}$) and to a greater degree than the alanine aminotransferase (ALT; see Section 10.7), but the most notable feature is usually a marked (five-fold or greater) elevation of the serum gamma-glutamyl transpeptidase (GGTP). Markedly elevated GGTP activities can be seen even when there are only mild abnormalities in the other LFTs and, for this reason, it was thought for a time that the GGTP was a useful marker of heavy alcohol consumption. However, it is now known that a *normal* GGTP does not exclude alcoholic liver disease and this, together with the susceptibility of this enzyme to induction by xenobiotics (Chapter 9) and the fact that equally disproportionate increases in its activity are seen in other conditions (e.g. malignancies not necessarily involving the liver, see Chapter 8), reduces its value as an indicator of alcohol abuse.

In patients with *alcoholic fatty liver* or *inactive cirrhosis*, any of the above parameters (individually or in combination) may be abnormal, but equally often they may all be normal. The finding of an increased AST as the sole abnormality in the absence of signs or symptoms of liver disease is most frequently associated with fatty liver due to obesity, whether or not the latter is related to alcohol.

Hypoalbuminaemia and hyperglobulinaemia are common findings but protein electrophoresis is generally of little value in the diagnosis of alcoholic liver disease because the serum protein changes are so variable. However, determination of the serum concentrations of the different immunoglobulin classes is recommended (see Section 10.6.4).

There is a fairly widespread opinion that patients with alcoholic cirrhosis have low (< 30–$35\,g\,l^{-1}$) serum albumin concentrations and that the finding of a normal serum albumin tends to reduce the likelihood of underlying cirrhosis but this is based on studies in patients who were hospitalized for decompensated cirrhosis (Chapters 1 and 2). In our experience, the vast majority of out-patients with well-compensated, biopsy-proven alcoholic cirrhosis have serum albumin concentrations within the normal range.

10.6.2.2 Other biochemical parameters

Other helpful biochemical findings include hypercholesterolaemia with or without hyperlipidaemia. Episodes of hypoglycaemia are not uncommon, particularly in patients in poor nutritional state, while hyperglycaemia and impaired glucose tolerance may be related to chronic pancreatitis (a common complication of alcoholic liver disease). Alcoholic ketoacidosis is also relatively common, particularly among women who drink heavily, and there is often a lacticacidaemia. Hypokalaemia due to renal potassium loss is also a fairly frequent finding and may be accompanied by low serum calcium and magnesium concentrations.

Abnormal iron storage is a common complication of prolonged heavy alcohol intake [14]. With certain notable exceptions, e.g. the Bantus of southern Africa (see Chapter 11), this does not seem to be due to increased dietary intake of iron, but is possibly related to some effect of alcohol on the regulation of iron absorption from the gut which is still not clearly understood [15]. Biochemical evidence of increased body iron stores in heavy drinkers includes elevations in serum iron and ferritin concentrations. Although of little value in screening for alcoholic liver disease [16], these two parameters should be measured and, if abnormal, should be further investigated to exclude underlying idiopathic haemochromatosis (Chapter 11).

A more specific parameter, namely the ratio desialylated to fully sialylated transferrin in the serum [18], may prove to be of value especially when there is no history of excessive alcohol intake. This ratio has been shown to be increased two- to 13-fold in persons consuming more than 100 g of alcohol per day (whether or not there is underlying liver damage), but is not altered in other conditions so far studied [19]. However, despite attempts to simplify the technique [19], the specific measurement of desialylated serum transferrin is still a relatively cumbersome procedure and is at present available in only a few specialist laboratories.

Serum glutamate dehydrogenase is said to be a more reliable marker of hepatocellular necrosis in alcoholic liver disease than are the other liver enzymes, but this view is not universally held. It has also been suggested that measurement of the serum activity of the mitochondrial isoenzyme of AST provides a highly sensitive (> 70%) and specific (> 80%) test for chronic alcohol abuse, with a positive predictive value of about 90% [17], but this has not been independently confirmed.

10.6.3 Haematology

Macrocytosis (with or without anaemia) is probably the most frequent haematological finding in alcoholic patients and is generally more marked than in other forms of liver disease. Plasma vitamin B_{12} and folate levels are usually low, even in patients who are apparently well nourished. The erythrocyte sedimentation rate (ESR) and mean corpuscular volume (MCV) are usually increased. Leucocyte counts are seldom normal. Leucopenia may be observed, but more often there is a pronounced leucocytosis which can present a difficult problem in the differential diagnosis from microbial infections (see Section 10.7). Other findings include anaemia, thrombocytopenia and a mildly prolonged prothrombin time, but these abnormalities are variable.

10.6.4 Immunology

Measurement of the serum immunoglobulin concentrations can be very helpful. The serum IgA concentration is elevated in about 80% of patients with alcoholic liver disease — much more frequently and more markedly than in other liver disorders — and is reportedly [20] related to the histological severity of the underlying lesion. The serum IgG concentration may also be moderately raised (to about 20 or $25\,g\,l^{-1}$) in those with hepatic parenchymal inflammation but usually to a lesser extent than is seen in other conditions such as autoimmune chronic active hepatitis (Chapter 6). IgM concentrations are usually normal or only slightly elevated.

Circulating autoantibodies are not normally associated with alcoholic liver disease but an autoantibody screen should be requested to exclude other liver disorders. However, the results will depend on the age of the patient and the nature of the alcohol-induced liver damage. Thus, older patients may well be seropositive for ANA and/or SMA at titres up to 1 : 80 and those with active cirrhosis are likely to be anti-LSP positive (Chapter 6). If facilities are available for measuring "anti-alcohol" antibodies, these may also be helpful (see Section 10.5).

10.6.5 Urinalysis

As a general rule, urinary abnormalities will be related to the severity of the condition and are not specific to alcoholic liver disease, although increased urinary potassium is worthy of comment because it is associated with hypokalaemia (see above) and urate concentrations are often low (with hyperuricaemia) due to lacticacidaemia.

Perhaps the most useful urinary parameter is the coproporphyrin concentration. Alcohol induces delta-aminolaevulinic acid synthetase and this leads to increased production of coproporphyrin, which is excreted in the urine. Since other conditions in which coproporphyrinuria occurs are relatively rare (see Chapter 11), the finding of increased coproporphyrin levels in urine should raise the question of alcohol abuse.

10.7 Differential diagnosis

As noted above, alcohol-related liver disorders share many clinical and laboratory features with other liver conditions, which must be excluded. This is particularly important when a history of excessive alcohol consumption is obtained, because the latter may be only incidental to some other (possibly treatable) underlying condition.

Alcoholic hepatitis must be distinguished from acute viral hepatitis. Thus, a viral screen should be requested (Chapter 5). If the patient is seronegative for markers of hepatitis A and B infection, the possibility of an acute non-A non-B hepatitis should be considered (Chapter 5). Perhaps the most useful parameters in this situation are the serum AST and the alanine aminotransferase (ALT). In acute viral hepatitis of any aetiology, the ALT is customarily increased to the same or, more often, to a greater extent than the AST, giving an AST : ALT ratio of 1 or 1 : 2. In alcoholic hepatitis the reverse is usually found, with the AST being characteristically increased to a greater extent than the ALT at ratios of 2 : 1 to 5 : 1 (see Table 10.2).

Since several of the chronic liver diseases (particularly chronic active hepatitis of various aetiologies; Chapter 6) can present acutely, these must also be excluded. An autoantibody screen should be requested (see above and Chapter 6) and the appropriate tests to exclude haemochromatosis and Wilson's disease should be performed (see Chapter 11). Furthermore, in addition to the viral screen, it may be considered appropriate to test for evidence of other microbial infections (Chapter 12).

References

1. Goldberg SJ et al. Gastroenterology 1977; 72: 598.
2. Levin DM et al. Am J Med 1979; 66: 429.
3. Pequignot G et al. Int. J Epidemiol 1987; 7: 113.
4. Saunders JB et al. J R Soc Med 1984; 77: 204.
5. Saunders JB and Williams R. Br Med J 1983; 287: 1819.
6. Montiero E et al. Hepatology 1988; 8: 455.
7. Bailey RJ et al. Br Med J 1976; 2: 727.
8. Morgan M et al. J Clin Pathol 1980; 33: 488.
9. Popper H and Lieber CS. Am J Pathol 1980; 98: 695.
10. Crapper RM et al. Liver 1983; 3: 327.
11. Lewis KO and Paton A. Lancet 1982; ii: 188.
12. Crossley IR et al. Gut 1986; 27: 186.
13. Hoerner M et al. Hepatology 1988; 8: 569.
14. Chapman RW et al. Dig Diseases Sci 1982; 27: 909.
15. Mazzanti R et al. Alcohol and Alcoholism 1987; 22: 47.
16. Chick J et al. Alcohol and Alcoholism 1987; 22: 75.
17. Nalpas B et al. Hepatology 1986; 6: 608.
18. Stibler H et al. Acta Med Scand 1979; 206: 275.
19. Storey EH et al. Lancet 1987; i: 1292.
20. Van de Wiel et al. Gastroenterology 1988; 94: 457.

Suggested further reading

Crapper RM, Bhathaland PS and Mackay IR. Chronic active hepatitis in alcoholic patients. Liver 1983; 3: 327–337.

Goldberg SJ, Mendenhall CL, Connell AM and Chedid A. "Non-alcoholic" chronic hepatitis in the alcoholic. Gastroenterology 1977; 72: 598–604.

Jenkins W. Liver disorders in alcoholism. Contemp Issues Clin Biochem 1: 258–270.

Levin DM, Baker AL, Riddell RH, Rochman H, Boyer JL. Non-alcoholic liver disease. Overlooked causes of liver injury in patients with heavy alcohol consumption Am J Med 1979; 66: 429–434.

MacSween RNM. Alcohol and liver injury: genetic and immunological factors. Acta Med Scand 1984; 703: 57–65.

McGregor RR. Alcohol and immune defense. JAMA 1986; 256: 1474–1479

Neuberger J, Williams R. Immunology of drug and alcohol-induced liver disease. In: Baillière's Clinical Gastroenterology, Vol. 1, No. 3 (Wright R and Hodgson HJF, Eds). London: Baillière Tindall, 1987: 707–722.

Pettersson G. Liver alcohol dehydrogenase. CRC Crit Rev Biochem 1987; 21: 349–389.

Ryback RS, Eckhardt MJ, Felsher B and Rawlings RR. Biochemical and haematological correlates of alcoholism and liver disease. JAMA 1982; 248: 2261–2265.

Shaper AG, Pocock SJ, Ashby D, Walker M and Whitehead TP. Biochemical and haematological response to alcohol intake. Annals Clin Biochem 1985; 22: 50–61.

Sorensen TIA, Orholm M, Bentsen K, Hoybye G, Eghoe K and Christoffersen P. Prospective evaluation of alcohol abuse and alcoholic liver injury in men as predictors of development of cirrhosis. Lancet 1984; ii: 241–244.

Van de Wiel A, Schuurman HJ and Kater L. Alcoholic liver disease: An IgA-associated disorder. Scand J Gastroenterol 1987; 22: 1025–1030.

11

Metabolic liver disorders

11.1   Introduction

There is a very large number of inherited disorders that either directly or indirectly affect the liver. Individually most of these conditions are quite rare, but collectively they comprise a significant proportion of liver disease worldwide. They range from diseases associated with excessive tissue storage of iron (haemochromatosis) or copper (Wilson's disease), through abnormalities of carbohydrate, lipid and amino acid metabolism, to defects in bilirubin excretion. Many present in early childhood and constitute a major part of paediatric liver disease. For this reason, a discussion of biliary atresia (not strictly speaking a metabolic disorder but important in the differential diagnosis of "neonatal hepatitis") is included here. It is essential to diagnose these disorders when they occur, because many are treatable and several can have disastrous consequences if appropriate management is not initiated promptly.

Although definitive diagnosis requires specialist expertise in some of the conditions, most of the disorders are associated with characteristic findings on laboratory investigation that should raise the level of suspicion in a patient with evidence of liver disease.

11.2   Iron-storage diseases

Excessive deposition of iron in the liver and other tissues occurs in a

TABLE 11.1. Conditions other than primary idiopathic haemochromatosis that may be associated with elevated serum iron concentrations

---

Acute hepatic necrosis

Acute iron intoxication (rare)

Anaemias
    Acute haemolytic
    Megaloblastic
    Sideroachrestic

Cirrhosis (especially alcohol induced, see Chapter 10)

Erythroleukaemia

Pancytopenia

Porphyria cutanea tarda (see Section 11.5.3)

Secondary iron overload (see Section 11.2.2)
    Dietary (Bantus)
    Oral iron supplementation
    Multiple blood transfusions

Thalassaemia

---

wide range of conditions and may not always be of primary pathological significance (Table 11.1). The term *haemochromatosis* (HC) is used to describe a group of disorders in which the excess iron causes parenchymal tissue damage and the group is subdivided according to whether the condition is primary, *idiopathic* (genetic) HC, or is related to some other aetiological factor, i.e. *secondary* HC, but there is a tendency to describe the latter group of conditions as *secondary iron overload* to enhance the distinction from primary idiopathic HC (IHC).

11.2.1 Idiopathic haemochromatosis

This is a genetic disorder with an autosomal recessive mode of inheritance of a gene located on the short arm of chromosome 6. This gene is in close proximity to the HLA A locus and is linked with inheritance of the HLA antigen A3. Linkages with other HLA allotypes, notably B7 and B14, have been described, but their significance is uncertain. If untreated, the accumulation of iron in hepatocytes and Kupffer cells causes chronic liver damage, leading to the development of cirrhosis which progresses fairly rapidly with fatal consequences. Treatment (phlebotomy at weekly or fortnightly intervals, usually for at least two years, until iron stores are depleted) dramatically improves prognosis [1].

The standard biochemical liver function tests (LFTs) are not very helpful in the diagnosis of IHC. The results are often only mildly abnormal and give no real indication of the nature of the underlying disorder. The main diagnostic problem relates to the differentiation of IHC from alcoholic liver disease (Chapter 10 and Sections 11.2.1.2. and 11.2.2), because a history of excessive alcohol consumption is not uncommon in IHC patients. Very occasionally, IHC can present as chronic active hepatitis (Chapter 6), but confusion with this condition is rarely a problem if the appropriate tests are performed (see below).

11.2.1.1 Diagnostic tests for IHC

Specific tests for body iron stores must be requested (Table 11.2). Most routine laboratories will report on the serum iron concentration and the total iron binding capacity (TIBC) of the serum. In the normal individual, the serum iron concentration ranges from 10 to $30 \, \mu mol \, l^{-1}$ ($55-170 \, \mu g \, dl^{-1}$) and the TIBC is about $45-70 \, \mu mol \, l^{-1}$ ($250-390 \, \mu g \, dl^{-1}$). The difference reflects the fact that the iron transport protein *transferrin* is normally only about one-third saturated. The degree to which the transferrin is saturated is calculated by expressing the serum iron as a percentage of the TIBC.

The serum iron, on its own, is not very informative because up to a quarter of patients with iron overload have values within the normal range and, conversely, it is not uncommon for healthy individuals to have levels in excess of $30 \, \mu mol \, l^{-1}$. Transferrin saturation is almost always $> 50\%$ and often $> 60\%$ in untreated IHC, but the false-positive rate is also high (about 30%). Most authorities agree that the serum concentration of the iron-storage protein, *ferritin*, is the best index of both hepatic and total body iron stores and the development of reliable radioimmunoassay (RIA) and enzyme-linked immunosorbent assay (ELISA) techniques for serum ferritin measurement has led to the availability of this test in many routine laboratories. The normal serum ferritin concentration is $< 200 \, \mu g \, l^{-1}$. In IHC, most patients will have levels of $> 1000 \, \mu g \, l^{-1}$, but, very occasionally, results within the normal range may be found.

TABLE 11.2. Typical laboratory findings in idiopathic haemochromatosis (IHC) and secondary iron overload[a]

	Symptomatic IHC	Asymptomatic IHC	Secondary iron overload
Liver function tests	Mildly abnormal	Normal	Variable
Serum iron ($10-30\ \mu mol\ l^{-1}$)	Usually >30	>30, but often normal	Usually >30
TIBC ($45-70\ \mu mol\ l^{-1}$)	Usually normal	Normal	Normal, very occasionally >70
Transferrin saturation ($20-50\%$)	>50% often >60%	>50%	Usually >60% often normal
Serum ferritin ($<200\ \mu g\ l^{-1}$)	>>500, often >5000	>500, often >1000	Usually <500, often normal

[a] Normal ranges shown in parentheses. TIBC, Total iron-binding capacity.

Measurement of the concentration of transferrin in serum (as distinct from calculation of the transferrin saturation level) is not very helpful. Hypotransferrinaemia can occur as a primary defect, associated with iron-refractory sideropenic anaemia and increased hepatic iron storage, or may be secondary to infections, malignancy or protein-losing enteropathies but, in IHC, transferrin concentrations are usually within the normal range ($1\cdot5-3\cdot4\ g\ l^{-1}$) and the occasional abnormalities are too variable to be of value in diagnosis.

Patients with IHC are usually seronegative for most autoantibodies other than occasionally low titres of ANA and/or SMA, depending on age. However, screening for autoantibodies and for microbial infections should be undertaken to exclude other disorders (see Chapters 5, 6 and 12).

11.2.1.2 Hepatic iron and total body iron stores

If the serum tests indicate markedly increased body iron stores, the diagnosis should be confirmed by liver biopsy. Appropriate staining of the sections will reveal the excessive deposition of iron in hepatocytes and Kupffer cells, but a quantitative measurement of the liver iron content should also be made. Normal liver usually contains less than 1 mg (18 μmol) of iron per gram dry weight. In IHC, the hepatic iron concentration is generally in excess of 10 mg g^{-1} (180 μmol g^{-1}).

Total body iron in the average IHC patient is about 20–40 g (360–720 mmol), compared with 2–4 g in normal individuals. The serum ferritin concentration bears a fairly linear relationship with mobilizable iron stores (1 μg l^{-1} of serum ferritin is approximately equivalent to 8 mg of body iron [2, 3]) and can be used as a guide to iron depletion while the patient is undergoing venesection therapy.

The recommended aim of phlebotomy in IHC is to bring the serum ferritin concentration down to the normal range and the serum iron to below 150 μg dl^{-1} (27 μmol l^{-1}). The serum iron begins to fall only when available iron stores are depleted (see Fig. 11.1) and this can be used to distinguish between patients with IHC and those with alcoholic liver disease who have evidence of iron accumulation (when

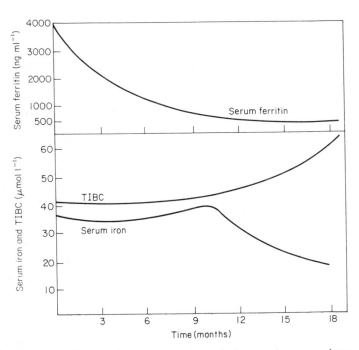

FIG 11.1.   Schematic representation of changes in serum iron parameters in idiopathic haemochromatosis during phlebotomy therapy.

there may be doubt about the diagnosis). In the latter case, iron deficiency will usually become apparent after only about one to two months of venesection, whereas in IHC at least one to two *years* is required for iron depletion.

11.2.1.3 Screening for asymptomatic IHC

Because treatment so effectively improves prognosis, early diagnosis of IHC is essential. First-degree relatives of patients with IHC are at particular risk of developing the disease and initiation of phlebotomy therapy as soon as there is evidence of iron accumulation, and before this begins to cause tissue damage, is considered important. Screening for HLA A3 is expensive and requires the services of a specialized laboratory. In addition, the association of A3 with IHC is not as strong as some of the HLA-linkages in other disorders, for only about 75% of IHC patients have A3 and this allotype is present in about 30% of the normal population. Tissue typing is therefore of little practical clinical value (although it can be useful for distinguishing between homozygous and heterozygous relatives once the haplotypes of the proband have been identified).

The serum ferritin and the transferrin saturation are the most widely used non-invasive screening tests for pre-cirrhotic IHC. The serum ferritin level begins to rise when hepatic iron stores reach about twice normal and at this stage the transferrin saturation will be > 50%. However, caution should be exercised in the interpretation of these tests when they are used for screening purposes. Persistently elevated serum ferritin and transferrin saturation levels, together, are strongly suggestive of increased hepatic iron stores and should be confirmed by liver biopsy (see Section 11.2.1.2), but mild increases in serum ferritin often occur in the absence of iron overload. This is particularly the case in patients with hepatocellular necrosis (e.g. in acute hepatitis or in toxic liver injury) and in subjects who are consuming excessive amounts of alcohol. Conversely, IHC patients who are deficient in ascorbic acid (which affects iron mobilization) may show falsely low results of these tests of iron status. On the other hand, normal individuals who are taking vitamin-C supplements may show evidence of elevated iron stores. With these reservations, the transferrin saturation and serum ferritin tests are reliable for screening purposes [3].

11.2.1.4 Dynamic tests

Among the dynamic methods that have been employed as screening tests, the old Fishback skin test [4] (involving intradermal injection of

Prussian blue) is no longer used. The *desferrioxamine infusion test* is, however, still occasionally applied. This involves the intramuscular injection of $0\cdot5\,g$ of desferrioxamine (other iron-chelators have also been used) and measurement of urinary iron excretion during the following 24 h. Under these conditions, total urinary iron excretion in IHC patients almost always exceeds $3\cdot0\,mg$ (normal $< 1\cdot5\,mg$) and is often $> 8\cdot0\,mg$ per 24 h. However, the test measures only chelatable iron and is of little value in diagnosing asymptomatic, pre-cirrhotic IHC.

11.2.1.5   Associated conditions

IHC is frequently associated with other conditions, some of which may be the eventual cause of death and all of which can contribute significantly to morbidity and may mask the diagnosis. These include diabetes mellitus (a very common presenting feature), hypogonadism (testicular atrophy, gynaecomastia and loss of libido; see Chapter 7), cardiomyopathy (usually in the later stages of IHC) and arthropathy. Appropriate investigations should be performed to identify or exclude these associated conditions in order that therapy may be instituted where indicated. In addition, because hepatocellular carcinoma is a complication of cirrhosis due to IHC as frequent as in cirrhosis of other aetiologies, periodic estimations of serum α-fetoprotein (AFP) should be made (Chapter 8).

11.2.2   Secondary iron overload

A proportion of patients with cirrhosis (due to causes other than IHC) will show some increased deposition of iron in the liver. This may be accompanied by increased serum iron and modest elevations of serum ferritin and, occasionally, of the transferrin saturation, but these changes are very rarely of the magnitude seen in IHC (Table 11.2). Although such abnormalities may be found in cirrhosis of any aetiology, they are most common in alcoholic liver disease and particularly in males with porphyria cutanea tarda (see Section 11.5.3).

   The reason for the association of iron overload with alcoholism is unclear. It may be due to enhancement of iron absorption from the gut by alcohol or it may be related to pancreatic insufficiency or to folic acid deficiency (see Chapter 10). The latter is a common finding in alcoholic patients, giving rise to a folate-deficiency anaemia, and it is important to exclude prescribed or self-administered oral iron supplementation as the cause of any serum abnormalities of iron status that may be detected. In general, however, dietary iron overload is rare, with the notable exception of the Bantus of southern Africa, who develop a syndrome similar to IHC that is related to consumption of alcoholic beverages brewed in iron pots.

Other conditions in which secondary iron overload is a feature include the haemolytic anaemias (particularly those due to ineffective erythropoiesis) associated with thalassemia major, congenital spherocytosis and the hereditary sideroblastic and sickle-cell anaemias. Secondary iron overload is also common in individuals receiving multiple blood transfusions, e.g. chronic renal dialysis patients, but in contrast to the iron loading related to ineffective erythropoiesis (which is predominantly parenchymal) parenterally acquired iron tends to be loaded into reticuloendothelial cells. As with cirrhosis, iron overload in these disorders may be associated with mild elevations in serum ferritin and transferrin saturation levels.

For any of the above conditions, underlying IHC must be suspected if the serum ferritin concentration rises above $1000\,\mu g\,l^{-1}$ and the transferrin saturation level exceeds 50%. It is important to make this distinction, because phlebotomy therapy (which is of such benefit in IHC) is ineffective in most secondary iron overload disorders and is often contraindicated.

11.3 Copper-storage diseases

Abnormal accumulation of copper in the liver and other tissues occurs in one well-documented genetic disorder (Wilson's disease) and in a number of acquired conditions. The main non-invasive tests for copper metabolism are of the serum and urinary copper and the serum concentration of ceruloplasmin. The latter is a blue copper-containing glycoprotein that is synthesized by the liver and is found in normal serum at a concentration of $13-27\,\mu mol\,l^{-1}$ ($200-400\,mg\,l^{-1}$). Its function is not fully understood but it appears to play an important role in regulating the level of copper in the body.

11.3.1 Wilson's disease

Wilson's disease is an inborn error of metabolism that leads to abnormal deposition of copper, first in the liver and then progressively in the kidneys, brain, eyes and other tissues. Accumulation of copper in the eyes is associated with the appearance of Kayser–Fleischer rings in the cornea (detectable by slit-lamp examination) and accumulation in the brain leads to the development of well-recognized neuropathology. The Wilson's disease gene has a worldwide distribution and is inherited as an autosomal recessive trait with a prevalence of 1 : 200,000 for homozygotes and 1 : 200 for heterozygotes. The disease affects older children (usually > 3 years) and younger adults (< 50 years), with a peak of onset in adolescence and only the occasional homozygote remaining healthy until the sixth decade [5].

The liver manifestations vary widely in presentation, from the silent development of cirrhosis to a more acute onset that may resemble acute viral hepatitis, chronic active hepatitis or (in older subjects) alcoholic liver disease and may rapidly progress to fulminant hepatic failure (Chapters 5, 6 and 10). Accurate diagnosis is essential, for this is a serious, life-threatening condition and early institution of treatment with copper chelators (D-penicillamine being the agent of choice) may be very effective for arresting or preventing the development of cirrhosis and reversing the neurological symptoms.

In view of the above, *it is considered essential that Wilson's disease be excluded in any young person with evidence of chronic liver disease.*

Initial laboratory findings will depend on how the disease presents. With an insidious onset, routine LFTs may show a mild increase in serum aminotransferase activity as the sole abnormality or there may also be modest elevations of the cholestatic indices (Table 11.3). When the disease presents more acutely, marked derangement of the LFTs (indicating hepatocellular damage) will be observed. In fulminant Wilson's disease, it has been noted [6] that haemoglobin concentrations and serum aminotransferase activities are lower, and serum bilirubin levels higher, than in fulminant hepatic failure (FHF) due to other causes. However, it is doubtful whether such comparisons are helpful in diagnosing Wilson's disease in the individual patient.

Wilson's disease presenting as chronic active hepatitis (CAH) can be confused initially with CAH of other aetiologies. Patients should be screened for the hepatotrophic viruses (Chapter 5) and for serum autoantibodies (Chapter 6). Occasionally, low titres of antinuclear (ANA) and/or smooth muscle (SMA) antibodies may be found and this can lead to a misdiagnosis of autoimmune CAH (AI-CAH). In the absence of ANA and SMA and of evidence of a viral aetiology, the differential diagnosis is from the subgroup of autoantibody-negative, presumed autoimmune (AI) CAH patients who are corticosteroid responsive and from non-A, non-B (NANB) virus infection. In our

TABLE 11.3. Typical laboratory findings in Wilson's disease[a]

| | Wilson's disease | | |
| | Symptomatic | | |
	Insiduous onset	Acute onset (fulminant)	Asymptomatic
Liver function tests	Abnormal but variable (Section 3.1.1)	Severely deranged	Usually normal
Serum copper			
Total ($10–30\,\mu mol\,l^{-1}$)	Variable	>30	Variable
Free ($<2\,\mu mol\,l^{-1}$)	>10	>10	>2
Serum ceruloplasmin ($13–30\,\mu mol\,l^{-1}$)	<13	<13	<20
Urinary copper ($0\cdot25–0.75\,\mu mol$ per 24 h)	>2	>15	>1
Hepatic copper ($<1\,\mu mol$/per g dry wt.)	>4 often >10	>4 often >10	$1–4$
Dynamic tests			
Radiocopper incorporation	Very low	Not known	Low
D-Penicillamine test (see Section 11.3.1.3)	>20-Fold increase in urinary copper	Not known	>10-Fold increase in urinary copper

[a] Normal ranges shown in parentheses.

experience, patients with Wilson's disease are almost always seronegative for anti-LSP and anti-ASGP-R autoantibodies (Chapter 6) and this distinguishes them from AI-CAH patients, whether or not the latter are seropositive for ANA and SMA. This does not, however, exclude NANB infections (in which anti-LSP and anti-ASGP-R also rarely occur).

11.3.1.1 Diagnostic tests for Wilson's disease

The diagnosis of Wilson's disease requires assessment of copper status (Table 11.3). Measurement of serum ceruloplasmin concentration is the blood test of choice. About 95% of homozygous Wilson's patients have serum ceruloplasmin concentrations of less than $13\,\mu\text{mol}\,l^{-1}$ ($20\,\text{mg}\,dl^{-1}$) and the rest have levels below $20\,\mu\text{mol}\,l^{-1}$, i.e. at the lower end of the normal range (Table 11.3). Hypoceruloplasminaemia also occurs in about 10% of Wilson's disease heterozygotes.

Urinary copper should also be measured. In almost all patients with symptomatic Wilson's disease, urinary copper excretion is at least three-fold higher than the normal rate of $0\cdot25$ to $0\cdot75\,\mu\text{mol}\,\text{day}^{-1}$ ($15-45\,\mu\text{g}\,\text{day}^{-1}$). Although it is customary also to measure total serum copper concentrations, the results may not be helpful. Some 90% ($10-25\,\mu\text{mol}\,l^{-1}$; $60-150\,\mu\text{g}\,dl^{-1}$) of the copper in normal serum is bound irreversibly to ceruloplasmin. The remainder ($< 2\,\mu\text{mol}\,l^{-1}$) is loosely bound to albumin and to amino acids. The latter, termed the "free" copper fraction, may be elevated 10-fold or greater in Wilson's disease but this increase is often masked by the profound decrease in ceruloplasmin-bound copper. Thus, total serum copper concentrations may be normal or even lower than normal.

Caution must be exercised, however, when interpreting results of any of the above tests in patients with evidence of severe hepatocellular necrosis (i.e. markedly elevated serum aminotransferase activities and/or prothrombin times). Because ceruloplasmin is synthesized by the liver, any condition in which overall hepatic synthetic function is impaired may lead to temporary reduction of serum ceruloplasmin concentrations [7]. Also, because the normal route of copper excretion is via the bile, severe hepatic necrosis in a patient with a long-standing cholestatic disorder (see Section 11.3.2.2) will cause release of stored copper from the liver and lead to high serum and urinary copper concentrations.

In fulminant Wilson's disease [6], urinary copper excretion may exceed $50\,\mu\text{mol}\,\text{day}^{-1}$ ($3\,\text{mg}\,\text{day}^{-1}$), i.e. 100 times normal. This parameter is also increased in FHF due to other causes, but not to the same extent (usually $< 15\,\mu\text{mol}\,\text{day}^{-1}$). Serum ceruloplasmin concentrations are generally lower in FHF due to Wilson's disease than that of other aetiologies but there is considerable overlap between individual patients (Tables 11.3 and 11.4). In this situation, the most discriminatory test may be the total serum copper concentration, which is always elevated ($> 30\,\mu\text{mol}\,l^{-1}$; $180\,\mu\text{g}\,dl^{-1}$) in fulminant Wilson's disease but is low ($< 15\,\mu\text{mol}\,\text{l}^{-1}$) in other FHF patients (if the latter condition is not superimposed on a chronic cholestatic disorder).

11.3.1.2 Hepatic copper

If any of the above tests shows a marked abnormality, a liver biopsy should be performed and the copper content determined. The normal hepatic copper concentration is less than $1\,\mu\text{mol}$ ($60\,\mu\text{g}$)/g dry weight of liver. In untreated patients with Wilson's disease, the hepatic copper content is almost always at least four times higher ($> 4\,\mu\text{mol}\,\text{g}^{-1}$) and may be increased 40- or 50-fold. However, the copper is not uniformly distributed throughout the liver and very occasionally values of $2\text{--}4\,\mu\text{mol}\,\text{g}^{-1}$ may be found as a result of sampling error. Values in this range may be seen in heterozygotes carrying one of the Wilson's disease genes but almost never exceed $4\,\mu\text{mol}\,\text{g}^{-1}$. Values above $4\,\mu\text{mol}\,\text{g}^{-1}$ *together with* a serum ceruloplasmin concentration of less than $13\,\mu\text{mol}\,\text{l}^{-1}$ are found only in patients with Wilson's disease.

11.3.1.3 Dynamic tests

In the absence of a liver biopsy, or if results of the above tests are inconclusive, either of two dynamic tests may be applied (Table 11.3). One of these involves the measurement of the rate of clearance of radioactive copper [8]. The latter is given as an oral dose and, normally, is rapidly taken up by the liver where it is incorporated into newly synthesized ceruloplasmin, which is then exported to the blood. This can be documented by monitoring the radioactive copper levels in plasma over the following three or four days. Heterozygotes for Wilson's disease show diminished incorporation of radiocopper into ceruloplasmin and homozygotes (whether or not symptomatic) show virtually no incorporation.

A simpler dynamic test involves measurement of urinary copper excretion before and after D-penicillamine administration. Urine is collected for a 24-h period and stored. An oral dose of $0\cdot5\,\text{g}$ of D-penicillamine is then given and urine collection recommenced. Twelve hours later a second dose of $0\cdot5\,\text{g}$ of the drug is given and urine collection continued up to the end of the second 24-h period. The total copper excreted during the two periods is then determined. A 20-fold increase after D-penicillamine is considered to be virtually diagnostic of Wilson's disease.

11.3.1.4   Monitoring D-penicillamine therapy

Some 20% of patients receiving D-penicillamine can be expected to exhibit sensitivity reactions to the drug. These usually develop within the first fortnight of treatment and the clinical signs are often accompanied by a leucopenia and thrombocytopenia. Because of this and of the need to assess the efficacy of the treatment, it is customary to monitor patients twice weekly for the first two months, monthly for the next 6 to 12 months and at extended intervals thereafter. In addition to the standard LFTs, full blood counts should be performed on each occasion along with urinalysis (including copper estimation). The latter is advisable not only to monitor the decrease in copper excretion as hepatic copper stores become reduced, but also for the early detection of proteinuria (or exacerbation of pre-existing proteinuria) which can herald the development of D-penicillamine induced nephrotic syndrome or Goodpasture's syndrome [9].

11.3.1.5   Other abnormalities

Leucopenia, thrombocytopenia and a coagulopathy are often seen in Wilson's disease. Haemolytic anaemia may contribute to jaundice and is a bad prognostic sign. A prognostic index based on the serum aminotransferase activity, the bilirubin concentration and the prothrombin time has been derived [10]. Other abnormal laboratory findings relate mainly to copper induced renal damage, which is common in untreated patients. Renal tubular acidosis, aminoaciduria, glycosuria, hypercalciuria, phosphaturia (with hypophosphataemia), proteinuria, and uricosuria (with hypouricaemia) are frequent findings.

11.3.1.6   Screening for asymptomatic Wilson's disease

Because early institution of D-penicillamine therapy is so effective for arresting the progress of this serious disorder, it is considered essential to screen all first-degree relatives for underlying (asymptomatic) Wilson's disease and advisable to also screen second-degree relatives. Urinary and serum copper, serum ceruloplasmin and standard LFTs should be performed (Table 11.3). Of these, the serum ceruloplasmin concentration is the most reliable and if this is less than 13 μmol l^{-1} the hepatic copper content should be determined. It is advisable to measure hepatic copper and/or perform one of the above two dynamic tests also when serum ceruloplasmin concentrations are found to be at the lower end of the normal range (i.e. $< 20\,\mu\mathrm{mol\,l}^{-1}$) *and* either the urinary or serum copper levels are greater than twice normal.

11.3.2 Secondary copper overload

11.3.2.1 Indian childhood cirrhosis

Excess oral intake of copper, even when ingested in gross quantities (e.g. with suicidal intent), rarely leads to serious hepatotoxic effects. A major exception may be *Indian childhood cirrhosis* (ICC), in which a high copper intake (from natural sources or from milk that has been stored in copper vessels) by genetically susceptible individuals has been implicated [11], but this is still the subject of debate. ICC is a severe and usually fatal liver disorder that affects children under 10 years of age, with a peak onset at between one and three years. It is confined to certain parts of Asia, notably Pakistan, Bangladesh, India, Sri Lanka, Malaysia and Burma, but is occasionally seen in Asian immigrant communities in other countries [12].

Routine LFTs show marked abnormalities indicating hepatocellular necrosis with a variable degree of cholestasis. The serum immuno-globulins are usually elevated and smooth-muscle antibodies are found in up to half of the patients. Thus, depending on how it presents clinically, ICC can be confused with acute viral hepatitis (Chapter 5) or autoimmune chronic hepatitis (Chapter 6). There is, as yet, no information on the occurrence of liver autoantibodies in ICC, but a viral aetiology can be excluded by the appropriate tests (Chapter 5). However, the latter are not always helpful because the hepatitis viruses are endemic in areas where ICC is most common and concomitant infection may mask the diagnosis.

Assessment of copper status may reveal elevations in serum and urinary copper, but these abnormalities rarely approach those seen in Wilson's disease (Table 11.4). The differential diagnosis from Wilson's disease is straightforward because serum ceruloplasmin concentrations are normal in ICC, except in the advanced stages of the disease when hepatic synthetic function may be impaired to an extent where ceruloplasmin levels begin to fall. Definitive diagnosis requires the finding of characteristic histological features on liver biopsy [13] and determination of hepatic copper content. In ICC, the latter is usually intermediate between the levels found in asymptomatic and symptomatic Wilson's disease.

TABLE 11.4. Typical laboratory findings relating to copper status in conditions other than Wilson's disease.[a]

	Acute hepatic necrosis	Chronic cholestasis	Indian childhood cirrhosis
Serum copper			
Total ($10-30\,\mu\text{mol}\,l^{-1}$)	> 15	>25	>25
Free ($<2\,\mu\text{mol}\,l^{-1}$)	<2	<2	<2
Serum ceruloplasmin ($13-30\,\mu\text{mol}\,l^{-1}$)	8–20	13–30	13–30
Urinary copper ($0\cdot25-0\cdot75\,\mu\text{mol per }24\,\text{h}$)	Usually <15	>1	>0·75
Hepatic copper ($<1\,\mu\text{mol/g dry wt}$)	<1	Usually >2 often >10	1–4

[a] Normal ranges shown in parentheses.

11.3.2.2 Other conditions

Since copper is normally excreted in the bile, any intra- or extra-hepatic interference with bile flow will lead to accumulation of copper in the liver. In chronic cholestatic conditions (e.g. primary biliary cirrhosis) this can be quite marked and may even be greater than that seen in Wilson's disease (Table 11.4). In addition, it can be accompanied by elevations in serum and urinary copper concentrations. However, in contrast to Wilson's disease, serum ceruloplasmin concentrations are always normal or even slightly elevated, except when there is concomitant severely diminished hepatic synthetic function that may lead to temporary reduction of ceruloplasmin levels.

11.4 α1-Antitrypsin deficiency

α1-Antitrypsin (α1AT) is a protease inhibitor (Pi) that occurs normally in serum at a concentration of $2-5\,\text{g}\,l^{-1}$. Deficiency of this protein is associated with pulmonary emphysema and often with liver disease. In Caucasians (see below), α1AT deficiency accounts for up to 15% of non-infectious hepatic disorders in children (it is a major consideration in the differential diagnosis of neonatal hepatitis; see Tables 11.8 and 11.9) and young (< 30 years) adults, but is also found in older individuals. The liver disease may be insidious, presenting late as a cryptogenic cirrhosis, but it can present more acutely as CAH and must be distinguished from CAH due to other causes (see Chapter 6).

α1AT is a glycoprotein which is synthesized mainly by the liver and deficiency states are related to genetically determined amino acid point substitutions in the protein moiety and/or defects in glycosylation that inhibit export of the glycoprotein from liver cells to the blood. The defective glycoprotein accumulates in the liver where it can be demonstrated histologically as PAS (periodic acid-Schiff) positive, diastase resistant granules in hepatocytes.

The concentration of α1AT in blood is determined by two alleles on chromosome 14 in close proximity to the gamma-globulin heavy-chain gene. Inheritance is autosomal and the alleles are codominant, i.e. each controls the production of one type of α1AT independently of the other allele in the chromosome pair. Worldwide, at least 26 different alleles have been described and the variations in amino acid sequences coded for by these alleles and the resulting alterations in glycosylation lead to production of α1AT molecules that differ in their isoelectric points and, consequently , in their electrophoretic mobility. The conventional nomenclature defines individual phenotypes by the letters Pi followed by an alphabetical code that describes the electrophoretic mobility of the α1AT produced by the particular allele. PiM (medium) is the commonest allele, occurring in about 90% of all populations studied, and individuals who are homozygous for M (PiMM) have normal serum concentrations of α1AT (Table 11.5). Of the other alleles, the most frequent are the PiS (slow) and PiZ (ultraslow) and individuals with these alleles have lower serum α1AT concentrations. A rare variant, Pi_{nul} (Pi−), is associated with no detectable α1AT in serum.

Population studies have revealed significant variations in the frequencies of certain phenotypes in different ethnic groups. The homozygous Z phenotype (PiZZ) is found most often among caucasoids of north-western European extraction, while the PiS allele is commonest among Iberians. In contrast, both of these alleles are extremely rare in negroes, North American Indians, Australasian aborigines and in Middle Eastern populations. Liver disease is commonest in PiZZ homozygotes, but the mechanisms involved in hepatic injury are poorly understood.

α1AT deficiency can be revealed by routine serum protein electrophoresis (Chapter 3), for the glycoprotein comprises about 90% of the normal $α_1$-globulin band which may be consequently markedly

TABLE 11.5. Approximate frequencies of α-1-antitrypsin (α1AT) phenotypes in European caucasoid populations and their relationships to serum α1AT concentrations and clinical liver disease

Phenotype (Pi)	Approximate frequency (%)	Serum α_1AT concentration (% of normal)	Liver disease in	
			Children	Adults
MM	90	100	0	0
MS	5	60	?	?
MZ	3	60	+ +	+ +
SS	1	60	?	+
FZ	0·02	60	?	+
SZ	0·2	40	+ +	+ +
ZZ	0·05	15	+ + +	+ + +
Z_{nul}	0·01	10	+	?

?, No data available; + + +, established association; + +, often reported; +, occasionally reported; 0, no association

reduced. However, this change may be noticeable in only the most severely α1AT-deficient subjects and is often masked by the increase in the total globulin fraction that accompanies the liver disease. Accordingly, more precise methods for α1AT measurement are required. This may be achieved by determining the trypsin inhibitory effect of the serum, but most routine laboratories now measure specific α1AT serum concentrations by radial immunodiffusion, by immunoelectrophoresis or by nephelometry (see Technical Notes, Chapter 6).

Since α1AT is one of the acute-phase reactants (Chapter 6), its serum levels may be artificially increased in response to inflammatory stimuli (e.g. in acute or chronic liver disease), even in α1AT-deficient subjects. Certain drugs may also increase α1AT concentrations. On the other hand, artificially low levels may occur in patients with severe acute hepatic necrosis or with protein-losing enteropathies. With these reservations, the diagnosis can usually be made on the basis of the serum α1AT concentrations. Where there is doubt, the issue can also be resolved by determining the phenotype of the individual and, if necessary, also of family members.

Phenotyping [14] is most commonly performed by examining the electrophoretic patterns of serum α1AT after acid starch gel electrophoresis and crossed immunoelectrophoresis, but isoelectric focusing (electrophoretic separation according to isoelectric point in pH gradient polyacrylamide gels) is being used increasingly. However, these techniques will require the services of a specialized laboratory where adequate reference sera and the necessary expertise for interpretation are available.

Abnormalities in the standard biochemical LFTs vary with the underlying hepatic pathology. Neonates with liver disease due to α1AT deficiency may show a markedly cholestatic picture, with a severe conjugated hyperbilirubinaemia, which is indistinguishable from that seen in biliary atresia (Section 11.9.9). Patients presenting with CAH due to α1AT deficiency will show biochemical changes typical of those associated with CAH due to other causes (Chapters 2 and 6).

11.5 Porphyrias

The porphyrias are a group of hereditary or acquired disorders of haem metabolism that lead to abnormal production of porphyrin and other precursors of haem synthesis. Most, if not all, of the hereditary and some of the acquired porphyrias are associated with skin lesions related to photosensitivity.

The liver and bone marrow are the main sites of haem synthesis and each type of porphyria is related to a specific enzyme defect that affects either the liver or the bone marrow but not both. Of those that affect the liver (Table 11.6), *protoporphyria* and *porphyria cutanea tarda* occur fairly frequently and may be associated with severe liver disease. Clinical presentation is very variable.

The results of routine laboratory tests depend on the type of porphyria and its presentation and whether the patient already has liver disease of some other aetiology. Diagnosis requires identification of the specific metabolic defect (Table 11.6) and is important, because treatment will depend on the type of porphyria and the condition may be exacerbated by exogenous agents, including alcohol and a wide range of drugs, which should be avoided. However, the techniques for establishing the nature of the defect are fairly specialized and many are not generally available in routine laboratories.

TABLE 11.6. Porphyrias affecting the liver

Type	Enzyme defect	Principal laboratory features
Protoporphyria	Ferrochelatase	High blood and faecal protoporphyrin and coproporphyrin. Normal urinary porphyrins. Erythrocytes show red fluorescence under UV light
Acute intermittent porphyria	Uroporphyrinogen I synthetase	High urinary ALA and porphobilinogen
Coproporphyria	Coproporphyrinogen oxidase?	High urinary ALA and porphobilinogen. High faecal coproporphyrin
Variegate porphyria	Protoporphyrinogen oxidase. Ferrochelatase?	High urinary ALA and porphobilinogen. High faecal protoporphyrin
Porphyria cutanea tarda	Hepatic uroporphyrinogen decarboxylase?	Normal urinary ALA and porphobilinogen. High urinary uroporphyrin I and coproporphyrin I. Elevated serum iron, ferritin and transferrin saturation

ALA, δ-aminolevulinic acid

11.5.1 Protoporphyria

Liver disease in this condition usually presents with a cholestatic pattern of biochemical LFTs but may progress rapidly to fulminant hepatic failure with the typically gross derangement of these parameters. In less severe cases, other routine laboratory findings are unremarkable. In particular, the haemoglobin concentration is often normal or only slightly reduced.

The laboratory diagnosis is fairly straightforward. Patients have high levels of protoporphyrin in the blood, often exceeding $1 \, mg \, dl^{-1}$ (or $50-100 \, \mu g \, dl^{-1}$ in plasma), and circulating erythrocytes (mainly reticulocytes) will show a characteristic evanescent red fluorescence when examined under light of approximately 400-nm wavelength. High concentrations of protoporphyrin are also found in the stools, but urinary porphyrins are normal. Coproporphyrin levels are often moderately increased in blood and faeces.

11.5.2   Haem-deficient hepatic porphyrias

This group of three disorders, *acute intermittent porphyria* (AIP), *hereditary coproporphyria* (HCP) and *variegate porphyria* (VP), is characterized by three distinct enzyme defects with an autosomal dominant mode of inheritance that lead to a potential reduction of hepatic haem synthesis and are associated with overproduction of δ-*aminolevulinic acid* (ALA). All are highly sensitive to alcohol and to a wide range of drugs (e.g. barbiturates, phenothiazines) that induce cytochrome P450 (Chapter 9) and any of which may precipitate acute attacks. AIP is much more common in Caucasians than in Negroes or Orientals. VP has a worldwide distribution, but is particularly prevalent among South Africans of Dutch ancestry, while HCP tends to be latent and is the rarest of the three.

Unless there is concomitant liver disease of some other aetiology, routine LFTs usually show a modest increase in serum amino-transferase activity as the main abnormality. The blood film is unremarkable, with a normal leucocyte count or occasionally a mild leucocytosis with a normal differential cell count. Among the other laboratory findings, hypercholesterolaemia and hyponatraemia are not uncommon and total serum thyroxine levels are often elevated. The latter is due to increased thyroid-binding globulin (Chapter 7), other thyroid function tests being normal.

The most striking finding in some patients is dark urine, which may vary in colour from wine-red to brownish (rapidly darkening on standing, particularly in sunlight) and which must be distinguished from the orange–brown colour in hyperbilirubinuria associated with other liver disorders. Even when the urine is not obviously abnormally coloured, urinary porphobilinogen (and its precursor, ALA) will be elevated in all three hepatic porphyrias. This can be demonstrated by the Watson–Schwartz test using Ehrlich's reagent, which forms a pink complex with porphobilinogen that remains in the aqueous phase after extraction with chloroform or butanol; this is in contrast to other substances (e.g urobilinogen) in urine which form red compounds with Ehrlich's reagent that are extractable with organic solvents. A modification, the Hoesch test [15], obviates the need for organic solvent extraction and may be simpler to perform.

ALA excretion is a less reliable indicator of these conditions because urinary levels are also increased in hereditary tyrosinaemia (Section 11.7) and in cases of heavy metal intoxication.

11.5.3 Porphyria cutanea tarda

Porphyria cutanea tarda (PCT) is probably the commonest porphyria seen in Caucasians. It is a haem-compensated porphyria that has a predilection for males and often occurs in association with liver disorders due to other causes, particularly in relation to excessive alcohol consumption, which exacerbates the condition. In females, it may be associated with oestrogens in contraceptive preparations. In contrast to the haem-deficient porphyrias, acute attacks are not precipitated by inducers of cytochrome P-450 (other than alcohol and oestrogens) and excretion of ALA and porphobilinogen is normal.

The results of routine LFTs will depend on whether there is an associated liver disorder of some other aetiology and are generally not very informative. On the other hand, serum iron concentrations are usually elevated and serum transferrin saturation may be increased to 60% or greater. In PCT patients with active liver disease, the serum ferritin concentration is also increased and these abnormalities are accompanied by increased deposition of iron in the liver, which can be depleted by phlebotomy. This overall picture may lead to confusion with idiopathic haemochromatosis (IHC) (Section 11.2.1), with which there appears to be a link. However, the changes in parameters of iron status are not as marked as in symptomatic (homozygous) IHC and PCT can be conclusively differentiated (from other porphyrias as well as from IHC) by the finding of high concentrations (often exceeding 1 μmol per 24 h (800 μg per 24 h)) of uroporphyrin I as well as coproporphyrin I in the urine.

11.5.4 Screening for carriers of porphyria

The value of screening family members varies with the type of porphyria. Symptomatic homozygotes are rare and most patients and asymptomatic carriers appear to be heterozygotes. Why the diseases should manifest themselves in some such individuals and not in others is unclear, but this suggests that exogenous precipitating factors (e.g. drugs, alcohol) may be required. With some porphyrias, the screening techniques are relatively straightforward and knowledge that an individual is a carrier is important to warn against exposure to exogenous initiating factors but, with others, the screening assays are so highly specialized and demanding (and the benefits so minimal) that they are hardly worthwhile.

The simplest screening test for carriers of protoporphyria involves examining peripheral blood erythrocytes for the characteristic red fluorescence at 400 nm (Section 11.5.1 and Table 11.6). For HCP, elevated faecal coproporphyrin and, for VP, increased faecal protoporphyrin is highly suggestive. About 70% of carriers of AIP have raised urinary porphobilinogen concentrations but a negative result is not exclusive. If there is doubt, assays for the specific enzyme defects will be needed to resolve the issue, but these will require the services of a specialized laboratory. With PCT, the defective enzyme appears to be *hepatic* uroporphyrinogen decarboxylase but the assay for this enzyme is difficult to perform and, because a relatively small proportion of carriers develop the condition and this is readily treated, screening is usually not considered justified.

11.5.5 Secondary porphyrinuria

Mild to moderate increases in urinary uroporphyrin and/or coproporphyrin without concomitant elevations of ALA or porphobilinogen are seen in a wide range of hepatic (viral hepatitis, toxic liver injury, hereditary conjugated hyperbilirubinaemia, Dubin–Johnson syndrome) and non-hepatic (Hodgkin's disease, haemolytic anaemia, leukaemia, myocardial infarction) disorders. The main significance of these abnormalities relates to the need for an awareness of their common occurrence in order to avoid misdiagnosis of one of the hereditary porphyrias. However, this benign coproporphyrinuria can be useful in the differential diagnosis of hereditary conjugated hyperbilirubinaemia (Rotor's syndrome) and Dubin–Johnson syndrome (Sections 11.9.2 and 11.9.3). In the former, the ratio of the coproporphyrin isomers I and III in urine is about 3 : 2 (normally 1 : 4) while, in the latter, the ratio is increased to about 9 : 1.

11.6 Disorders of carbohydrate metabolism

11.6.1 Galactosaemia

This is a disorder in which deficiency of the enzyme galactose-1-phosphate uridyl transferase leads to accumulation of galactose-1-

phosphate, galactilol and galactose in all tissues, and to severe liver disease. The latter is reflected in the gross derangement of the routine LFTs, with a predominantly cholestatic picture but also with raised serum aminotransferases indicating hepatocellular necrosis. Other frequent laboratory findings include a prolonged prothrombin time, haemolytic anaemia, and aminoaciduria together with proteinuria indicating renal impairment.

A simple test for total reducing substances in urine should, if positive, raise the suspicion of galactosaemia and should be routinely performed in all children with signs or symptoms of liver disease. Specific (e.g. glucose oxidase based) tests for glucose should not be relied upon because the results are often normal in this condition. The definitive diagnosis of galactosaemia requires demonstration of absent or low galactose-1-phosphate uridyl transferase activity in erythrocytes. *The galactose tolerance test is not recommended*, as this may exacerbate the condition.

11.6.2 Fructosaemia

Three genetic defects in fructose metabolism have been identified: *Essential* (benign) *fructosaemia, hereditary fructose intolerance* and *fructose-1,6-diphosphatase deficiency.* The first of these is due to hepatic fructokinase deficiency and is not associated with any pathology. *Hereditary fructose intolerance* is related to a deficiency of the enzyme fructose-1-phosphate aldolase; it does not present a problem if dietary fructose is avoided but otherwise can lead to severe kidney and liver damage, in which event serum aminotransferases and bilirubin concentrations are markedly elevated, prothrombin time is protracted and these abnormalities are accompanied by hypoalbuminaemia, a profound hypoglycaemia, hyperaminoacidaemia, hypokalaemia, hypophosphataemia and a thrombocytopenia. The impaired renal function leads to aminoaciduria and proteinuria.

Fructose-1,6-diphosphatase deficiency usually has less severe effects on the liver. Serum aminotransferase activities are mildly or moderately elevated but, in contrast to hereditary fructose intolerance, serum bilirubin concentrations are at most only mildly increased. The prominent features are hypoglycaemia, lactic acidaemia, aminoacidaemia (particularly alanine and glutamine) and a marked ketoacidosis (which may occur in the absence of hypoglycaemia). In many respects the condition resembles some types of glycogen storage disease (see below); in particular, blood glucose concentrations do not rise following intravenous glucagon. The diagnosis of both this disorder and of hereditary fructose intolerance requires that a deficiency in the respective enzymes is demonstrated in liver biopsies.

11.6.3 Glycogen-storage diseases

Nearly a dozen distinct types and several sub-types of inherited

TABLE 11.7. Glycogen storage diseases

Type	Synonym	Tissue involved	Enzyme defect
0		Liver	Glycogen synthetase
I	Von Gierke disease	Liver, kidney, intestine	Glucose-6-phosphatase
II	Pompe's disease	All tissues	Lysosomal α-1,4- and α-1,6-glucosidase
III	Cori disease, Forbes disease, Limit dextrinosis	Liver, muscle, heart and other tissues	Amylo-1,6-glucosidase ($\pm$)-phosphorylase kinase
IV	Andersen disease, Amylopectinosis	Most tissues	Amylo-1,4-1,6-transglucosidase
V	McArdle syndrome	Skeletal muscle only	Muscle phosphorylase
VI		Liver only	Liver phosphorylase
VII		Skeletal muscle, erythrocytes	Phosphofructokinase
VIII		Liver, brain	Inactive liver phosphorylase ?
IX		Liver	Liver phosphorylase kinase
X		Liver, muscle	Cyclic-3,5-AMP-dependent kinase

disorders of carbohydrate metabolism leading to abnormal glycogen storage have been identified (Table 11.7). Most of these present in childhood and prognosis varies according to the type/sub-type from very poor (types II, IV and VIII) to good (types VI, VII and IX).

Routine LFT results in those types that affect the liver range from essentially normal to mildly cholestatic (jaundice is very rare), except in the later stages when liver failure (with the usual marked derangement of these parameters) leads to death. However, serum AST levels are usually moderately increased in types III, IV, VI, IX and X. A low fasting blood glucose concentration is the major finding and the hypoglycaemia may be a cause of mental retardation. In types I, III, VI and X, the response to intravenous glucagon (at a dose of $0 \cdot 7 \, \text{mg m}^{-2}$) is blunted, with blood glucose levels rising to less than $1 \cdot 9 \, \text{mmol l}^{-1}$ ($35 \, \text{mg dl}^{-1}$). In other types the response to glucagon is usually normal. Other frequent laboratory findings include hyperlipidaemia, acidosis and hyperuricaemia.

Clinical management depends upon knowledge of the type of glycogen storage disease. This requires identification of the specific enzyme defect(s) in the tissues. Among those that affect the liver, the defects can be identified in peripheral blood leucocytes from patients with types II, III, IV, VI or IX, but liver biopsies will be required for types O and I, and liver or muscle biopsies for type X.

11.7   Disorders of amino acid metabolism

The only genetically mediated disorder of amino acid metabolism that has so far been identified as a cause of significant liver disease is *hereditary tyrosinaemia*. Two types of this autosomal recessive condition are recognized: *type I* appears to be due mainly to deficiency of hepatic fumaryl acetoacetate hydrolase and is associated with a poor prognosis; and *type II* tyrosinaemia is due to deficiency of the cytosolic enzyme tyrosine aminotransferase and is not associated with liver damage.

Type I tyrosinaemia usually presents in early childhood with vomiting, diarrhoea, hepatosplenomegaly, ascites and failure to thrive. There is moderate to severe derangement of the LFTs (with a hyperbilirubinaemia of sufficient magnitude to cause jaundice in about 30% of patients) and a prolonged prothrombin time. The characteristic laboratory finding is a marked aminoacidaemia, with tyrosine, phenylalanine and methionine concentrations being particularly elevated. Serum α-fetoprotein (AFP) concentrations are usually elevated, sometimes quite markedly (up to about 100-fold). There is also a high concentration of succinyl acetoacetate in the urine and this is considered diagnostic.

Other findings relate to accompanying renal damage, leading to a renal tubular acidosis and associated with a generalized aminoaciduria, hyperphosphaturia (and hypophosphataemia) and glycosuria. The condition can be confused with fructosaemia (Section 11.6.2), from which it must be distinguished.

11.8 Lipidoses

There is a large number of inherited (autosomal recessive) disorders of lipid metabolism. Most present in early childhood and principally affect the central nervous system but almost all are associated with hepatomegaly, accompanied by (often severe) derangement of the LFTs, and death is frequently due to liver failure. Conjugated hyperbilirubinaemia is a common finding but is rarely of sufficient magnitude to cause jaundice, except terminally. Several of these disorders are associated with hyperlipidaemia and increased levels of free cholesterol in plasma, which may be suggestive. Diagnoses are usually made on clinical criteria together with demonstration of the specific enzyme defects.

11.9 Other disorders

In addition to the above, there are numerous other disorders of the liver in which genetic factors, or at least a genetic susceptibility to external agents, have been identified or are suspected. Some of these conditions are due to primary metabolic defects and others are secondary to anatomical abnormalities or to some other congenital disorder. Many are associated with hyperbilirubinaemia and often present in early childhood, comprising a significant proportion of the group of disorders that come under the general heading of "neonatal hepatitis", the differential diagnosis of which can be difficult and is highly specialized (Tables 11.8 and 11.9). Some, such as Gilbert's and the

TABLE 11.8. Some causes of pathological neonatal hyperbilirubinaemia

Unconjugated	Conjugated
Bacterial infection	Chromosomal abnormalities
Drugs	Drugs
Fructosaemia	Endocrine abnormalities
Galactosaemia	Haemolytic disease (severe)
Haemolytic disease	Hypoxia
Hypoglycaemia	Infections
Hypothyroidism	Inherited disorders (various)
Intestinal obstruction	Intravenous nutrition
	Vascular abnormalities

Crigler–Najjar syndromes and those that are secondary to endocrine abnormalities, have been covered elsewhere in this book (see Chapters 2 and 7) and this section deals with only a selection of the more extensively characterized conditions.

11.9.1 Benign recurrent intrahepatic cholestasis

This is a rare episodic cholestatic disorder that may affect several members of a single family. Onset is usually under the age of 30 years and the characteristic clinical features are malaise and lassitude with an intense pruritus (with or without an erythematous rash), which precede and continue throughout each episode of cholestasis.

Routine LFTs during one of these episodes show hyperbilirubinaemia, marked elevation (usually > 5-fold) of ALP, normal or only slightly raised serum GGTP and moderately elevated (< 5-fold) serum aminotransferases. Other parameters, including serum albumin and prothrombin time, are typically normal. At the start of an attack serum bilirubin levels may be normal, but serum bile acid concentrations are usually extremely high [16]. This contrasts with the situation in other forms of cholestasis, in which serum bile acids and bilirubin show parallel changes. Quantitative technetium-diisopropyliminodiacetic acid cholescintigraphy reportedly shows prompt uptake of the radionuclide, but no biliary excretion after 21 h [17]. However, too few patients have been studied to determine the diagnostic value of either this technique or of the serum bile acid/bilirubin ratios and the diagnosis is usually made on clinical

TABLE 11.9.   Recommended scheme of laboratory investigation of neonatal hepatitis[a]

Stage I: Blood	*Immediate investigations* Full blood count. Blood group (saving serum for cross-matching). Prothrombin time. Sugar, urea and electrolytes. Bacterial culture
Urine	Total reducing substances (**not** glucose alone) Bacterial culture Microscopic examination
Stage 2:	*Urgent investigations (i.e. as soon as practicable)* Biochemical LFTs (Chapter 2) including "direct" and "indirect" bilirubin α1-Antitrypsin serum concentration (Section 11.4), and phenotype (if appropriate) Full viral screen (Chapter 5) Screen for non-viral infection (Chapter 12), including WR or VDRL Autoantibody screen (Chapter 6) Coombs test (if appropriate) Erythrocyte galactose-1-phosphate uridyl transferase Serum and urinary amino acid concentrations Sweat electrolyte test
Stage 3	Percutaneous liver biopsy (reserving tissue for enzymatic analysis and microbial culture)
Stage 4	^{131}I-Rose-Bengal faccal excretion test (Chapter 2)

[a] Adapted from Mowat [18].

grounds, i.e. spontaneous resolution of symptoms and the serum abnormalities (which may last several months), and their recurrence at variable intervals.

11.9.2   Dubin–Johnson syndrome

This is a relatively rare condition characterized by both unconjugated and conjugated intermittent hyperbilirubinaemia and lysosomal deposits of

TABLE 11.10.   Principal laboratory features of various metabolic/congenital disorders that affect the liver

Disorder	Typical laboratory findings
α-1-Antitrypsin (α1AT) deficiency (Section 11.4)	Abnormal LFTs ranging from mild cholestatic to severe hepatocellular picture. Low serum α1AT
Benign recurrent intra-hepatic cholestasis (Section 11.9.1)	Episodic hyperbilirubinaemia, markedly elevated ALP, high serum bile acids, moderately elevated transaminases, normal or mildly abnormal serum GGTP, albumin and prothrombin time
Biliary atresia (Section 11.9.9)	Marked conjugated hyperbilirubinaemia. Acholic stools. Elevated ALP, GGTP, bile salts, etc. Serum transaminases may be mildly to moderately elevated
Byler's disease (Section 11.9.6)	Intermittent (becoming persistent) hyperbilirubinaemia. Markedly elevated serum transaminases and bile acids
Congenital hepatic fibrosis (Section 11.9.5)	Mildly to moderately increased ALP (also occasionally GGTP). Other LFTs normal
Criggler–Najjar syndrome (Chapter 2)	Severe progressive hyperbilirubinaemia. Serum bilirubin may reach $400-800\,\mu\text{mol}\,l^{-1}$ in type 1 (neonatal) but is usually about $100-400\,\mu\text{mol}\,l^{-1}$ in type 2 (older subjects)
Cystic fibrosis (Section 11.9.4)	Transiently elevated LFTs becoming more persistently abnormal. Conjugated hyperbilirubinaemia, hypoalbuminaemia
Dubin–Johnson syndrome (Section 11.9.2)	Intermittent mild to moderate hyperbilirubinaemia, other LFTs normal. High urinary urobilinogen and coproporphyrin I. Decreased urinary coproporphyrin III (I:III ratio about 9:1)
Fructosaemia (Section 11.6.2)	Variable with type but usually hypoglycaemia, ketoacidosis, hyperaminoacidaemia. Abnormal glucagon infusion test. LFTs mildly to grossly deranged.
Galactosaemia (Section 11.6.1)	Grossly abnormal LFTs. Increased total reducing substances in urine. Urinary glucose may be normal

TABLE 11.10. (*Continued*)

Disorder	Typical laboratory findings
Gilbert's syndrome (Chapter 2)	Intermittent mild (up to $100\,\mu mol\,l^{-1}$) hyperbilirubinaemia. Other LFTs normal
Glycogen storage diseases (Section 11.6.3)	Hypoglycaemia. Abnormal glucagon infusion test. LFTs vary with type from normal to mildly cholestatic, with usually moderately raised aminotransferases.
Haemochromatosis (Section 11.2.1)	Variable mildly to moderately abnormal LFTs. Raised serum iron and transferrin saturation. Markedly elevated serum ferritin.
Lipidoses (Section 11.8)	Moderate to gross derangement of LFTs, with predominantly hepatocellular pattern. High plasma lipids and free cholesterol
Mucopolysaccharidoses (Section 11.9.7)	Generalized mild to moderate abnormalities of LFTs. Dermatan, heparin and/or keratan sulphates in urine
Porphyrias Hepatic porphyrias (Section 11.5.2)	Mildly raised serum aminotransferases. Other LFTs usually normal or unremarkable. Raised urinary porphobilinogen and ALA
Porphyria cutanea tarda (Section 11.5.3)	Variable abnormalities of LFTs. Elevated serum iron, ferritin and transferrin saturation (but may be normal). High urinary uroporphyrin I and coproporphyrin I
Protoporphyria (Section 11.5.1)	Abnormal LFTs, mildly cholestatic but may become severely deranged. Protoporphyrin high in blood and stools but normal in urine. Moderately increased blood and stool coproporphyrins. Erythrocytes fluoresce at 400 nm
Reye's syndrome (Section 11.9.8)	Markedly elevated serum transaminases. Prolonged prothrombin time, hyperammonaemia, hypoglycaemia, electrolyte disturbances
Rotor's syndrome (Section 11.9.3)	Fluctuating predominantly conjugated, mild to moderate ($<170\,\mu mol\,l^{-1}$ hyperbilirubinaemia. Other LFTs normal. Urinary coproporphyrin I:III ratio about 3:2

continued

TABLE 11.10. (*Continued*)

Disorder	Typical laboratory findings
Tyrosinaemia (type I) (Section 11.7)	Moderate to gross derangement of LFTs, with predominantly hepatocellular pattern. Marked aminoacidaemia. Raised serum α-fetoprotein (AFP). High urinary succinyl acetoacetate.
Wilson's disease (Section 11.3.1)	Mildly to severely abnormal LFTs: pattern variable but aminotransferases usually elevated. Low serum ceruloplasmin. Raised urinary copper. Serum copper often elevated, but may be normal or even low

LFTs, Biochemical liver function tests; ALP, serum alkaline phosphatase; GGTP, serum gamma-glutamyl transpeptidase.

yellow–brown or black melanin-like pigment in hepatocytes that can be easily seen in liver biopsies. It has a worldwide distribution but is commonest in Arab races and in both Ashkenazic and Sephardic Jews. Patients are usually only mildly jaundiced or completely asymptomatic, the condition being revealed during routine screening or investigation of some other disorder. Occasionally, pregnancy or oral contraceptives may unmask the condition.

Routine LFTs are typically normal, apart from mild to moderately increased serum bilirubin concentrations. However, urinary levels of urobilinogen and coproporphyrin I are increased, and coproporphyrin III is decreased (see Section 11.5.5). Abnormal clearance of BSP, Rose-Bengal, methylene blue and ICG is a feature, but bile acids are excreted normally. The differential diagnosis is from Gilbert's syndrome (Chapter 2) and Rotor's syndrome (see below).

11.9.3 Rotor's syndrome

This benign, familial, chronic hyperbilirubinaemia was first described by Rotor in the Philippines. Serum bilirubin concentrations may fluctuate but are usually less than $170 \, \mu mol \, l^{-1}$ ($10 \, mg \, dl^{-1}$) and the conjugated pigment levels tend to be greater than those of the unconjugated. Other LFTs are normal.

The differential diagnosis is from Gilbert's (Chapter 2) and Dubin–Johnson (see above) syndromes. Unlike the latter, in Rotor's syndrome an oral cholecystogram will be normal and there is no pigment in hepatocytes. Cholephilic dye clearance kinetics are also quite different from those seen in Dubin–Johnson syndrome, from which Rotor's syndrome can also be distinguished by the ratios of coproporphyrin isomers I and III in the urine (Section 11.5.5).

11.9.4   Cystic fibrosis

Hepatobiliary abnormalities of varying severity (usually mild) are a fairly common and well-recognized complication of cystic fibrosis. In the majority of cases, there is excessive accumulation of lipid in hepatocytes, but there is no evidence that this leads to chronic liver disease. Occasionally, a prolonged conjugated hyperbilirubinaemia (due to extrahepatic biliary obstruction) together with severe hypo-albuminaemia is seen in infants with cystic fibrosis. As these children progress to adolescence, up to 20% may develop a biliary-type cirrhosis. Initially, transient elevations of ALP, GGTP and/or serum aminotransferases may be observed, but these parameters become more persistently abnormal as the cirrhosis progresses and the pro-thrombin time is frequently prolonged. A sweat electrolyte test should be performed to exclude previously unsuspected cystic fibrosis in children with idiopathic chronic liver disease (Table 11.9). Since children with cystic fibrosis are susceptible to all other forms of chronic liver disease, it is particularly important to exclude Wilson's disease (Section 11.3.1), other inherited disorders (see above) and autoimmune (Chapter 6) and microbial (Chapters 5 and 12) aetiologies in those with hepatic abnormalities.

11.9.5   Congenital hepatic fibrosis

This is a condition which is defined pathologically as the presence of bands of fibrous tissue joining portal tracts in the liver and often containing spaces lined by bile ducts. Portal hypertension is the major feature and the condition is often associated with renal disorders such as infantile polycystic disease. As in polycystic disease of the liver and kidneys, hepatocellular function seems not to be compromised and mild to moderate elevation of the ALP (and occasionally the GGTP) is often the only serum biochemical liver abnormality detected. The disorder must be distinguished from other forms of cirrhosis requiring different management. Diagnosis is usually made on the basis of the clinical findings together with assessment of a liver biopsy by an experienced histopathologist.

11.9.6 Byler's disease

This severe intrahepatic cholestatic disorder was first described in several members of an Amish family named Byler. Onset is usually within the first year of life but jaundice may be intermittent initially, becoming persistent later. LFTs are severely deranged with elevated serum aminotransferase activities, indicating hepatocellular necrosis, in addition to the hyperbilirubinaemia. Serum bile acids are also elevated, with lithocholic acid showing a preferential increase in some patients, but it is generally felt that these changes are not specific for this disorder.

11.9.7 Mucopolysaccharidoses

At least seven types of this group of acid mucopolysaccharide storage diseases have been identified. The diseases are associated with characteristic facies and hepatosplenomegaly is a common finding. Routine LFTs show generalized mild to moderate abnormalities. Diagnoses are based on the finding of dermatan, heparin or keratan sulphates in the urine and/or demonstration of the specific enzyme deficiencies in leucocytes.

11.9.8 Reye's syndrome

This is a disorder that affects children up to late adolescence. It usually follows a mild virus infection (typically influenza B or varicella) and is characterized by a severe encephalopathy with marked cerebral oedema but no significant inflammatory activity in the brain or meninges. It appears to be due to a severe metabolic disturbance arising from a gross (but reversible) abnormality of mitochondria, the underlying mechanism of which is unknown. There is marked accumulation of lipid in hepatocytes (and, to a lesser extent, in other organs), but liver-cell necrosis is usually minimal and, apart from hepatomegaly in a proportion of cases, there is seldom any clinical evidence of liver disease. Nevertheless, serum aminotransferase activities are markedly increased, prothrombin time is prolonged and hyperammonaemia, hypoglycaemia and electrolyte disturbances are frequently associated. It can be easily confused with several of the genetic disorders, particularly fructosaemia and cystic fibrosis, discussed above.

11.9.9 Extrahepatic biliary atresia

Biliary atresia is a severe, progressive, cholestatic condition of unknown cause that develops *in utero* or soon after birth. It is a life-threatening condition related to bile duct malformation and, although various palliative surgical procedures to relieve the biliary obstruction have shown beneficial effects in some cases (particularly when applied before 10 weeks of age), the only real "cure" seems to be liver transplantation. It presents a very real problem in differential diagnosis from other forms of neonatal jaundice, in which surgical intervention is often inadvisable.

The standard LFTs show a typically marked cholestatic pattern but are otherwise uninformative. Various authorities have suggested that serum α-fetoprotein, 5'-nucleotidase, GGTP, erythrocyte haemolysis in the presence of peroxidase, bile salt concentrations and ratios of the various bile salts are of value in diagnosis. Lipoprotein X, an abnormal low-density lipoprotein found in the sera of adults with extrahepatic biliary obstruction, has also been proposed as a useful marker in biliary atresia. However, others [18] have not found any of these parameters helpful and have suggested that often they may actually be misleading. Liver biopsy together with the ^{131}I-Rose-Bengal faecal excretion test have been suggested as the most useful diagnostic procedures [18]. The latter involves careful collection of stools (avoiding contamination with urine) during a 72-h period following intravenous injection of ^{131}I-Rose-Bengal dye. If excretion of the radiolabelled dye is less than 10% of the injected dose and the liver biopsy does not show features of hepatitis, Mowat [18] suggests that laparotomy should be considered (see also Chapter 2 and Section 10.6).

Acholic stools reflect the complete biliary obstruction in biliary atresia, but this can also be a feature in children with two other conditions that can present with a clinical picture similar to biliary atresia and in which surgical intervention is often beneficial, namely *choledocal cysts* and *spontaneous bile-duct perforation*. The latter is suggested by the finding of bile-stained ascites, but these two disorders cannot be easily distinguished from each other or from biliary atresia by the usual laboratory tests.

References

1. Bomford A and Williams R. Quart J Med (New Ser) 1976; 45: 611.
2. Brissot P *et al*. Gastroenterology 1981; 80: 557.
3. Bassett ML *et al*. Gastroenterology 1984; 87: 628.
4. Fishback HR. J Clin Lab Med 1939; 25: 98.
5. Fitzgerald MA. Mayo Clin Proc 1975; 50: 438.
6. McCullough AJ *et al*. Gastroenterology 1983; 84: 161.
7. Walshe JM and Briggs J. Lancet 1962; ii: 263.
8. Sternlieb I and Scheinberg IH. Gastroenterology 1979; 77: 138.
9. Sternleib I *et al*. Ann Intern Med 1975; 82: 673.
10. Nazer H *et al*. Gut 1986; 27: 1377.
11. Tanner MS *et al*. Lancet 1983; ii: 992.
12. Tanner MS *et al*. Br Med J 1978; 2: 928.
13. Tanner MS *et al*. Lancet 1979; i: 1203.
14. Talamo RC *et al*. Washington: DHEW Publ No (NIH) 78-1420, 1978.
15. Lamon J *et al*. Clin Chem 1974; 20: 1438.
16. Summerfield JA *et al*. Hepatogastroenterology 1981; 28: 139.
17. Minuk GY and Shaffer EA. Gastroenterology 1987; 93: 1187.
18. Mowat AP. Liver Disorders in Childhood, 2nd edn. London: Butterworths, 1987.

Suggested further reading

Bissell DM. Haem metabolism and the porphyrias. In: Liver and Biliary Disease, 2nd edn (Wright R, Millward-Sadler GH, Alberti KGMM and Karran S, Eds). London: Baillière Tindall, 1985: 387–413.
Bloomer JR. The liver in protoporphyria. Hepatology 1988; 8: 402–407.
Gollan JL. Editorial: Diagnosis of haemochromatosis. Gastroenterology 1983; 84: 418–421.
Javitt NB (Ed). Neonatal Hepatitis and Biliary Atresia. Bethesda: US DHEW Publication No. (NIH) 7-1296, 1979.
Mowat AP. Liver Disorders in Childhood, 2nd edn. London: Butterworths, 1987.
Nazer H, Ede RJ, Mowat AP and Williams R. Wilson's disease: Clinical presentation and use of prognostic index. Gut 1986; 27: 1377–1381.
Psacharopoulos HT and Mowat AP. The liver and biliary system. In: Cystic Fibrosis (Norman AP, Batten JC and Hodson ME, Eds). London: Baillière Tindall, 1983: 164–182.
Scheinberg IH and Sternlieb I. Major Problems in Internal Medicine, Vol. XXIII: Wilson's Disease. Philadelphia: WB Saunders, 1984.

Scott J, Gollan JL, Samourian S and Sherlock S. Wilson's disease presenting as chronic active hepatitis. Gastroenterology 1978; 74: 645–651.

Simon M and Brissot P. The genetics of haemochromatosis. J Hepatol 1988; 6: 116–124.

Talamo RC, Bruce RM, Langley CE *et al.* Alpha-1-antitrypsin laboratory manual. Washington: US DHEW Publication No. (NIH) 78-1420, 1978.

12

Granulomatous diseases and non-viral infections of the liver

12.1   Introduction

There is a large number of non-viral infections that either directly or indirectly involve the liver and several have been implicated as a cause of granulomatous liver disease. In areas where these infections are endemic clinicians will be aware that they are a major cause of hepatic disease, but in countries where they are less common they can be overlooked as a cause of biochemical liver abnormalities. Many of these conditions are related to what has previously been regarded as mainly tropical diseases, but with increasing travel and migration they are becoming more prevalent in temperate zones. A comprehensive discussion of such a multitude of disorders is beyond the scope of this book and this chapter merely summarizes the general laboratory findings in some of the more common conditions.

12.2   Granulomatous liver disease

Granulomata in the liver are seen in a very wide range of conditions (Table 12.1). They may be associated with acute hepatitic illnesses or with relatively inactive chronic liver disorders. With few exceptions, the standard biochemical liver function test (LFT) abnormalities are fairly unremarkable and are generally not very helpful. Diagnoses are usually based on liver biopsy findings in conjunction with identification of the primary disorder. The most frequent biochemical abnormality is an elevated serum alkaline phosphatase. Marked hyperbilirubinaemia is very rare and serum aminotransferase activities are normal or only slightly increased. In Europe and North America, the commonest causes of the granulomatous liver disease are *sarcoidosis* and *tuberculosis*. The latter, together with various other bacterial, as well as fungal and parasitic infections, are important in the tropics.

12.2.1   Sarcoidosis

Sarcoidosis is frequently associated with abnormalities of the biochemical LFTs but these are usually only mildly deranged. The most common finding is a moderate (three- to five-fold) increase in the serum alkaline phosphatase. Serum bilirubin concentrations are

TABLE 12.1   Some underlying causes of granulomatous liver disease

Idiopathic disorders	Infections
Chronic idiopathic granulomatous hepatitis	Bacterial
	Brucellosis
Crohn's disease	Leprosy
Erythema nodosum	Listeriosis
Hodgkin's disease	Mycobacterial
Polymyalgia rheumatica	Fungal
Primary biliary cirrhosis	Coccidioidomycosis
Sarcoidosis	Histoplasmosis
Ulcerative colitis	Parasitic
	Schistosomiasis
	Toxocariasis
	Rickettsial
Drugs	Spirochaetal
Aspirin	Viral
Chlorpropamide	Cytomegalovirus
Diazepam	Epstein–Barr virus
Hydralazine	
Methyldopa	
Penicillins	
Phenytoin	
Phenylbutazone	
Procainamide	
Quinidine	
Sulphonamides	
Thiazides	
Tolbutamide	

usually slightly elevated but jaundice is uncommon and marked increases in serum aminotransferase activities are rarely seen. Hyperglobulinaemia is frequent, with preferential increases in the serum immunoglobulins, especially IgG, although IgA and IgM concentrations may also be raised. Low titres of a variety of autoantibodies, including antinuclear (ANA) and/or antismooth muscle (SMA) antibodies (Chapter 6), can often be demonstrated along with high titres of a wide range of antibodies against common pathogens (e.g. Epstein–Barr virus, coliform bacteria, Rubella and *Mycoplasma*), reflecting a generalized heightened immunoresponsiveness. The disease has been reported to occur in conjunction with primary biliary cirrhosis [1].

There is no specific serological test for sarcoidosis. Diagnoses are based on a spectrum of clinicopathological findings including the involvement of the lungs and mediastinal lymph nodes. A positive Kveim–Siltzbach skin test is confirmatory. This involves intradermal injection of an extract of spleen tissue from a patient with active sarcoidosis. Development of a nodule at the site of injection within six weeks and demonstration of a typical granulomatous reaction upon biopsy of the nodule is considered a positive result. Although this test has a low false-positive rate (about 2%), only about 80% of patients with classical sarcoidosis are positive and the frequency of positive tests drops to less than 40% in those who do not have thoracic tissue involvement. This, together with the variability of the spleen-tissue extract preparations used for the test, has cast doubt on its reliability. Certainly, a negative Kviem test does not exclude sarcoidosis.

Serum activities of angiotensin-converting enzyme are elevated in cases of active sarcoidosis and this has attracted a great deal of interest as a possible gauge of disease activity, but this enzyme is of little value in diagnosing hepatic sarcoidosis because it is elevated in several other conditions including a number of liver disorders.

12.2.2 Tuberculosis

Hepatic granulomata are almost always found in acute miliary tuberculosis. In other forms of chronic tuberculosis, the incidence of liver involvement varies but is usually greater than 25%. This is often not clinically obvious, the illness presenting as pyrexia of unknown origin. In addition to increased serum alkaline phosphatase, hypoalbuminaemia, hypergammaglobulinaemia, leucocytosis and a high erythrocyte sedimentation rate are frequent but non-specific findings. Occasionally, massive liver involvement can lead to the formation of tuberculous abscesses (Section 12.3).

Diagnosis depends on a positive Mantoux skin test, but a negative test result does not always exclude tuberculosis.

12.3 Liver abscesses

Hepatic abscesses are broadly classified according to whether they are caused by bacterial (pyogenic abscesses) or amoebic infections (see below). As with the latter, pyogenic abscesses occur most frequently in older adults with biliary disease. When they do occur in the young, this is most often associated with systemic streptococcal or staphylococcal infections or, in neonates, with infections of the umbilicus. In adults, coliforms used to be the commonest organisms implicated, but it is now recognized that anaerobes and microaerophilic species and, particularly, *Streptococcus milleri* are more frequently associated with pyogenic liver abscesses (Table 12.2).

Identification of the responsible organism(s) can be difficult, partly because multiple infections are not uncommon [2, 3]. Current recommendations are that both aerobic and anaerobic blood cultures should be carried out *before* surgery is performed to drain the abscess (to avoid confusion due to peri-operative contamination or secondary infections) and the results should be correlated with the findings upon culture of the abscess material itself. Obviously, if antibiotic therapy is instituted before blood samples are taken for culture this will cloud the issue.

Whatever the cause of the abscess, the most frequently found biochemical abnormality is in the serum alkaline phosphatase activity, which can be quite markedly (five-fold or greater) raised, but serum bilirubin concentrations of $35-70 \, \mu\text{mol} \, l^{-1}$ are reportedly not uncommon (Table 12.3). Serum aminotransferase activities are usually near normal but may be raised by up to about three-fold and, in that event, are considered a bad prognostic sign. Hypoalbuminaemia and hypergammaglobulinaemia are frequent findings.

The haematological picture includes a marked leucocytosis, raised erythrocyte sedimentation rate (usually $> 100 \, \text{mm}^{-1}$), anaemia and (in protracted illnesses) prolongation of the prothrombin time.

The most important differential diagnosis of hepatic abscess is hepatocellular carcinoma and it is therefore worthwhile to measure the serum α-fetoprotein (AFP) (see Chapter 8). A high concentration will almost always indicate an underlying malignancy, but a negative result does not exclude hepatocellular carcinoma, because patients with such tumours may have normal AFP levels.

Among the other laboratory tests that might be performed, perhaps

TABLE 12.2 Some organisms that have been implicated as causes of pyogenic liver abscesses

Actinomyces	Mycobacteria
Aerobacter sp.	Pneumococci
Bacteroides	*Proteus* sp.
Clostridia	*Pseudomonas* sp.
Enterobacter sp.	*Salmonella*
Escherichia coli	Staphylococci
Klebsiella	Streptococci

TABLE 12.3 Typical laboratory findings in patients with hepatic abscesses

Test	Result
Biochemistry	
Alkaline phosphatase	Markedly elevated (usually five-fold or greater)
Bilirubin	Moderately elevated ($35\text{--}70\,\mu\text{mol}\,l^{-1}$)
Aminotransferases	Normal or only slightly raised
Albumin	Low
Globulins	Elevated
Haematology	
White-cell count	Marked leucocytosis
ESR	Markedly raised (usually $> 100\,\text{mm}\,h^{-1}$)
Haemoglobin	Low ($8\text{--}12\,\text{g}\,dl^{-1}$)
Prothrombin time	Slightly prolonged (INR < 2)
Recommended additional tests	
Serum α-fetoprotein	Within normal range
Serum vitamin B_{12}	High

the most useful is the serum vitamin B_{12}. High levels of vitamin B_{12} (often exceeding $1000\,\text{pg}\,ml^{-1}$) are very common in patients with hepatic abscesses, whereas normal or even low concentrations are found in patients with extrahepatic infections. The original bacteriological method for assaying serum B_{12} required five or six days to perform and the value of this parameter was therefore limited to some extent, but the development of a radioimmunoassay for the measurement of vitamin B_{12} has enhanced its usefulness in this context. However, a high vitamin B_{12} concentration is not specific for hepatic abscesses, for similar levels are seen in patients with malignant liver disease and in some other conditions.

12.4 Hepatic amoebiasis

Amoebic infections of the liver are much more common in tropical countries than in temperate zones. They may take the form of a hepatitic illness, "amoebic hepatitis", which is a poorly defined entity that must be distinguished from other forms of acute and chronic liver disease, or they may present as abscesses in the liver (see above). The latter are more frequently seen in older adults (they are very rare in young children) and most often they are secondary to long-standing biliary disease (whether or not this has been symptomatic).

Diagnosis relies on serology, i.e. the demonstration of IgM and IgG antibodies against the organism, for which there now exists a battery of tests including enzyme-linked (ELISA) and passive haemagglutination assays (see Section 6.9). Negative serology excludes amoebiasis but a positive test is not necessarily diagnostic of a current infection because this can simply be an indication of a previous exposure to the organism. Other laboratory findings in amoebic hepatitis are similar to those of acute hepatitis or chronic active liver disease generally (Chapters 2, 3 and 4). With amoebic abscesses, the findings are generally indistinguishable from those associated with other liver abscesses (Table 12.3) but the serum bilirubin is reportedly less often (and less markedly) elevated.

12.5 Leptospirosis

Leptospirosis is now relatively rare in Western Europe and in North America (about 50 to 100 cases per year) but sporadic outbreaks are not uncommon elsewhere in the world. It is caused by *Leptospira interrogans* organisms which are usually carried by rats and other feral mammals but domestic animals may also be hosts. Transmission is normally via animal bites or other close contact with the host animals. The illness usually follows a biphasic course and ranges from a mild febrile condition to a severe (often fatal) form characterized by deep jaundice. The jaundice is not secondary to hepatocellular necrosis, which is minimal. Rather, it appears to be related to impairment of bilirubin transport. This form of leptospirosis was thought to be almost always caused by *L. icterohaemorrhagiae* (when it is known as Weil's disease but other forms of Leptospira (notably *L. canicola*, carried by dogs) are now known to account for a significant proportion of cases.

12.5.1 Weil's disease

The most striking biochemical finding in this severe form of leptospirosis is a profound conjugated hyperbilirubinaemia with
bilirubinuria. The serum ALP is usually only moderately elevated and
serum aminotransferases are often normal or only slightly increased.
However, the ALP can be quite markedly raised and this picture may
lead to a misdiagnosis of extrahepatic biliary obstruction. In addition,
occasionally exceptionally high aminotransferase activities are found
and, because of the clinical features (fever, rashes, anorexia, malaise,
nausea, myalgia, etc.), the condition may be confused with acute viral
hepatitis.

There is usually a degree of renal impairment that may lead to renal
failure in some cases. Urinalysis reveals proteinuria, casts, and
increased numbers of erythrocytes and leucocytes. Uraemia may
develop, with blood urea concentrations rising to $20-40 \, \text{mmol} \, \text{l}^{-1}$
$(125-250 \, \text{mg} \, \text{dl}^{-1})$.

The main haematological finding is a leucocytosis. Cell counts as
high as $70\,000 \, \text{mm}^{-3}$ $(70 \times 10^9 \, \text{l}^{-1})$ have been documented. Anaemia
due to intravascular haemolysis frequently develops in the later stages
of the icteric disease and may be severe. Prothrombin times and
platelet counts are usually normal but hypoprothrombinaemia and
thrombocytopenia have been reported in some cases. Meningism is a
common feature and increased cell counts (up to $2000 \, \text{cells} \, \text{mm}^{-3}$) in
cerebrospinal fluid are frequently observed.

Diagnosis depends mainly on demonstrating antileptospiral antibodies in serum, for the organism itself appears in the blood only
during the early stages of infection. Specific tests for these antibodies
and for the precise serotype are available. The antibodies appear
during the second week of the illness and increase rapidly in titre over
the following three weeks. A four-fold rise in titre during this period is
usually considered as diagnostic. Thereafter, titres decline but the
patient may remain seropositive for several years.

12.6 Venereal diseases

Gonnorrhoea is very occasionally associated with a perihepatitis,
known as Fitz–Hugh–Curtis syndrome (which is more commonly
related to *Chlamydia* infections). Laboratory findings reflecting the

liver involvement may show a mild to moderate elevation in the serum aminotransferases as the sole abnormality, but are otherwise unremarkable and are usually not very helpful. The diagnosis is almost always made on the clinical findings (which, depending on the presenting features, can be confused with pleurisy or cholelithiasis) and demonstration of the infection.

Syphilis, and particularly congenital, secondary or tertiary syphilis, is a more common (but still relatively rare) cause of liver disease [4]. Liver function tests tend to show a mild to moderate, predominantly cholestatic, picture. The clinical features can be similar to those of viral hepatitis. Also, non-organ-specific autoantibodies are sometimes found in the serum and this can lead to confusion with the auto-immune liver disorders (Chapter 6).

12.7 Cestode infections

A number of cestode worms are capable of invading the liver. By far the most important are *Echinococcus* spp., of which *E. granulosus* is the commonest around the world. *E. multilocularis* and *E. oligarthrus* are also important. Liver disorders associated with *Taenia* infections (usually *T. saginata* or *T. solium*) are rare.

The tapeworms become trapped in the liver, almost always in the centrilobular veins of the right lobe, where they develop into fully encapsulated hydatid cysts. The differential diagnosis is from other cysts, from amoebic or pyogenic abscesses and from malignant or benign tumours. The manifestation is usually clinical, LFTs often being normal. However, as the hydatid cyst grows (at the rate of approximately 1 cm year^{-1}), compression of the surrounding liver tissue occurs. Depending on the precise location of the cyst, this can lead to mechanical obstruction of intrahepatic blood and bile flow resulting in congestion and cholestasis, with LFTs suggestive of extrahepatic biliary obstruction. Occasionally, there may be a super-imposed secondary infection or a cyst may rupture, leading to cholangitis and a reactive hepatitis with elevated serum amino-transferases.

Diagnosis depends on serology, for which there is a large number of tests available, including indirect haemagglutination, immunofluor-escence, immunodiffusion, complement fixation and radioallergosor-bent (RAST) tests, latex agglutination, electrophoretic immunossays and ELISA (see Section 6.9). The indirect haemagglutination method, developed in 1957, is still preferred. All these tests are subject to wide intra- and inter-laboratory variations and the current recommendation is that a combination of two or more tests should be employed.

12.8 Trematode infections

Trematode infections of the liver are exceedingly important in tropical and some sub-tropical areas. They are less prevalent in temperate zones but infections may remain dormant for many years and are therefore not uncommon among immigrant communities in non-endemic areas. Diagnosis can be difficult, because the hepatitis viruses are also endemic in the same areas and concurrent infections may serve to confuse. The main organisms involved are the blood flukes (*Schistosoma* sp.) and the liver flukes *Clonorchis*, *Fasciola* and, in certain parts of the Far East, *Opisthorchis* sp. Transmission is via faeces-contaminated fresh water in which snails breed that act as intermediate hosts, and infections are acquired by ingestion of cercariae through drinking the water or by eating vegetation or raw fish harvested from the contaminated water.

12.8.1 Schistosomiasis (Bilharzia)

Hepatic schistosomiasis is caused by *S. mansoni* or *S. japonicum*. The former is widespread, while the latter is mainly confined to certain parts of the Far East. The hepatic disease is due to a host immune reaction to ova deposited in the gut wall by the parasite and carried by the blood to the liver. Fibrosis is the dominant histological feature and is often severe but a picture closely resembling chronic active hepatitis is frequently seen.

The laboratory findings are very variable and depend on the stage of the disease (which may remain asymptomatic for many years). They range from only mild elevations in serum alkaline phosphatase and gamma-glutamyl transpeptidase to full-blown derangement of all the LFTs, including raised serum aminotransferase activities and hyperbilirubinaemia. Serum IgG concentrations are often increased and IgM to a lesser extent but IgA levels are usually normal. A variety of organ-specific and non-organ-specific autoantibodies (Chapter 6) has been reported [5] in the sera of schistosomiasis patients, but these appear to be of little diagnostic significance.

Diagnosis requires the microscopic demonstration of ova in stools and/or in liver and/or in rectal biopsies. A skin test may be used for screening purposes but this is prone to give false-positive results. A wide range of serological tests for schistosomal infections, including immunofluorescence, flocculation tests, complement fixation and other immunoassays, is available, but none is sufficiently reliable to replace direct demonstration of the parasite.

12.8.2   Liver flukes

These organisms colonize the biliary tract and the laboratory findings are those normally associated with large duct obstruction. The extent of the biochemical abnormalities depends on the stage of infection (which is often asymptomatic) and its severity. Anaemia is a common finding and a marked eosinophilia may be observed, especially in the early stages of *Clonorchis* infection. The latter predisposes to cholangiocarcinoma and is often associated with a pancreatitis, which may complicate interpretation of the laboratory findings. Skin tests and various serological tests for liver fluke infestations are available but their reliability is variable and, thus far, none replaces direct demonstration of parasite ova in stool specimens for definitive diagnosis.

12.9   Nematode infections

Although commonest in the tropics, nematode infections are worldwide and the worms sometimes invade the liver where they may cause liver abscesses (see above), cholecystitis (occasionally acute), pyogenic cholangitis and/or large duct obstruction. The main species involved are *Ascaris lumbricoides* (round worm), *Strongyloides stercoralis* and certain non-human parasites such as *Toxocara canis* and *T. catis*.

When there is invasion of the liver, the laboratory findings usually indicate mild to moderate cholestasis but more severe abnormalities may be observed according to the nature of the infection. Also, depending on the stage and severity of infestation, there may be a marked eosinophilia, iron-deficiency anaemia, generalized vitamin deficiency and other changes relating to the associated protein-losing enteropathy and, occasionally, pancreatitis.

12.10 Fungal infections

Fungal infections involving the liver are still seen fairly frequently in tropical areas but (with a few exceptions) in other countries hepatic involvement is mainly confined to immunocompromised individuals receiving intensive chemotherapy for malignancies or immunosuppressive treatment related to organ grafts or autoimmune diseases. Several are important causes of granulomatous liver disease (see Table 12.1). In many cases the diagnoses can be made by serological or skin tests, but in others histological demonstration of the infection is required and is often revealed only at autopsy.

12.10.1 Aspergillosis

Systemic infections, usually due to *Aspergillus fumigatus*, are relatively rare and liver involvement is uncommon [6]. However, aspergillosis has been associated with the Budd–Chiari syndrome, with markedly elevated serum bilirubin, ALP and aminotransferases [7].

12.10.2 Blastomycosis

This chronic systemic fungal disease is caused by *Blastomyces dermatitidis* (in North and South America) or by *Paracoccidioides brasiliensis* (mainly in Central and South America). The respiratory tract is the site of primary infection but hepatic involvement is seen in 20–50% of patients with disseminated disease [8–11]. Histological findings in the liver include granulomata, an inflammatory infiltrate, focal necrosis and occasionally fibrosis. The biochemical LFTs in these patients are often only mildly abnormal but can sometimes be severely deranged.

12.10.3 Candidiasis

Hepatic candidiasis [12] is particularly common in immunocompromised hosts [13] and is a major problem, especially in liver-graft recipients. *Candida* infection should be suspected in any immunocompromised individual with unexplained pyrexia, but it is important to note that only about half of those infected will have positive blood cultures. In the remainder, diagnoses require liver biopsies and all too often the diagnosis is made only at autopsy.

12.10.4 Coccidioidomycosis

This is an infection (usually confined to the respiratory tract) caused by *Coccidioides immitis*, which is endemic in South America and in south-western North America. Disseminated infection is relatively rare, but when it occurs up to 30% of patients will have hepatic involvement [14] with grossly deranged LFTs. Liver histology shows granulomata and an inflammatory infiltrate with focal necrosis and the condition can be confused with hepatic tuberculosis or sarcoidosis.

12.10.5 Cryptococcosis

Fungal infections due to *Cryptococcus neoformans* occur sporadically worldwide and are usually acquired through contact with domestic or wild animals (most frequently from bird droppings). Disseminated infection is rare but is usually associated with hepatosplenomegaly. LFTs are very variable but can be severely deranged and the condition has been misdiagnosed as sclerosing cholangitis [15].

12.10.6 Histoplasmosis

Systemic infection due to *Histoplasma capsulatum* is common in the USA. In chronic and in severe disseminated infection, hepatic involvement in the form of granulomatous hepatitis is common, but LFTs are very variable. The condition may be confused with sarcoidosis. Diagnosis depends on isolation and culture of the organism, usually from blood or bone marrow.

12.11 Q fever

Q fever is a flu-like illness caused by *Coxiella burnetti*, which is widely distributed in Europe and North America. Farm animals are the commonest source of infection. Hepatic involvement is well recognized but is usually asymptomatic and is often revealed only serendipitously by the finding of an elevated serum ALP. Occasionally, the serum aminotransferase activity may also be increased and in these cases confusion with viral hepatitis can arise. Histologically, the findings include a predominantly portal tract inflammatory infiltrate and granulomata with a characteristic ring of eosinophilic fibroid necrosis that is not always seen but, when found, is considered pathognomonic.

12.12 Systemic bacterial infections

Systemic bacterial infections can cause hepatic dysfunction even when the liver is not directly involved. Their importance in the present context relates to the likelihood that the hepatic abnormalities may distract attention from serious extrahepatic disease. In neonates and young children, a sudden and profound conjugated hyperbilirubinaemia (with serum bilirubin concentrations of up to $500\,\mu\mathrm{mol\,l}^{-1}$) can be the first evidence of a severe systemic infection, e.g. secondary to an *E. coli* urinary tract infection. Usually, this is the main (and often the only) biochemical liver abnormality.

In adults, a wide range of Gram-positive and Gram-negative organisms can cause jaundice, with serum bilirubin concentrations up to about $200\,\mu\mathrm{mol\,l}^{-1}$. These patients are usually very ill and the hyperbilirubinaemia will often be accompanied by a leucocytosis, normochromic anaemia and an elevated erythrocyte sedimentation rate. Hypoalbuminaemia and hypergammaglobulinaemia are common. Serum ALP activities may be raised, occasionally markedly so (up to 10-fold), in the absence of jaundice and may be the only liver abnormality detected. Serum aminotransferases are generally normal or only slightly elevated in these situations.

References

1. Keefe EB. Am J Med 1987; 83: 977.
2. Pitt HA and Ziudema GD. Surg Gynaecol Obstet 1975; 140: 228.

3. Sabbaj J *et al*. Ann Intern Med 1972; 77: 629.
4. Pareek SS. Dig Diseases Sci 1979; 24: 41.
5. Bassily S *et al*. J Trop Med Hyg 1973; 76: 153.
6. Varkey B. J Am Med Assoc 1983; 249: 2020.
7. Young RC. Arch Intern Med 1963; 124: 754.
8. Busey JF. Am Rev Resp Dis 1963; 89: 659.
9. Witorsch P and Utz JP. Medicine 1968; 47: 169.
10. Londero AT and Ramos CD. Am J Med 1972; 52: 771.
11. Teixeira F *et al*. Histopathology 1978; 2: 231.
12. Lewis JH *et al*. Hepatology 1982; 4: 479.
13. Tashjian LS. Rev Infect Dis 1984; 6: 689.
14. Bayer AS *et al*. Medicine 1976; 55: 131.
15. Lefton HB *et al*. Gastroenterology 1974; 67: 511.

Suggested further reading

Degremont A. Parasitic diseases of the liver. Baillière's Clinical Gastroenterology 1987; 1: 251–272.

Dunn MA and Kamel R. Hepatic schistosomiasis. Hepatology 1981; 1: 653–660.

Fauci AS and Wolff SM. Granulomatous hepatitis. In: Progress in Liver Diseases, Vol. 5 (Popper H and Schaffner F, Eds) New York: Grune & Stratton, 1976: 609–617.

Herzog C. Bacterial infections involving the liver. Baillière's Clinical Gastroenterology 1987; 1: 231–250.

Holdstock G, Balasegaram M, Millward-Sadler GH and Wright R. The liver in infection. In: Liver and Biliary Disease, 2nd edn (Wright R, Millward-Sadler GH, Alberti KGMM and Karran S, Eds). London: Baillière Tindall, 1987: 1077–1119.

Kagan IG and Maddison SE. Immunology of parasites: general aspects. In: Immunology of Human Infection. Part 2, Viruses and Parasites (Nahmias AJ and O'Reilly RD, Eds). New York: Plenum, 1982: 315–325.

Lewis JH, Patel HR and Zimmerman HJ. The spectrum of hepatic candidiasis. Hepatology 1982; 4: 479–487.

Moore-Gillon JC, Kykyn SJ and Phillips I. Microbiology of pyogenic liver abscess. Br Med J 1981; 283: 819–821.

Patterson M, Healy GR and Shabot JM. Serologic testing for amoebiasis. Gastroenterology 1980; 78: 136–141.

Romer FK. Angiotensin-converting enzyme activity in sarcoidosis and other disorders. Sarcoidosis 1985; 2: 25–34.

13

Reference values

The values given below are taken from several sources and are provided only as a guide. When assessing results of laboratory tests, **it is important to check the normal ranges of the laboratory that performed the tests.**

13.1 Blood

13.1.1 Physical values

pH, arterial	$7 \cdot 35 - 7 \cdot 45$
Plasma osmolality	$280 - 295 \, \mathrm{mOsm \, l^{-1}} \, (\mathrm{mmol \, kg^{-1}})$
Volume, blood	$50 - 80 \, \mathrm{ml \, kg^{-1}}$ body weight
Volume, plasma	$31 - 55 \, \mathrm{ml \, kg^{-1}}$ body weight

13.1.2 Cellular parameters

Erythrocyte sedimentation rate (ESR)	Male: $3-5\,\text{mm}\,\text{h}^{-1}$ Female: $4-7\,\text{mm}\,\text{h}^{-1}$
Haematocrit	See packed cell volume
Haemoglobin	See Section 13.1.5
Mean corpuscular volume (MCV)	$87-91\,\text{fl}\,(\mu^3)$
Packed cell volume (haematocrit)	Male: $40-54\%$ Female: $35-47\%$
Platelet count	$150-400 \times 10^9\,\text{l}^{-1}$ (or $\times 10^3\,\text{mm}^{-3}$)
Red-cell count	Male: $4\cdot5-6\cdot5 \times 10^{12}\,\text{l}^{-1}$ (or $\times 10^6\,\text{mm}^{-3}$) Female: $3\cdot9-5\cdot6 \times 10^{12}\,\text{l}^{-1}$
Red-cell diameter	$6\cdot7-7\cdot7\,\mu\text{m}$
Red-cell thickness	$1\cdot7-2\cdot5\,\mu\text{m}$
Red-cell volume	$23-35\,\text{ml}\,\text{kg}^{-1}$ body weight
Reticulocyte count	$0\cdot5-2\cdot0\%$ of red cells
White cell count	$4-11 \times 10^9\,\text{l}^{-1}$ (or $\times 10^3\,\text{mm}^{-3}$)
Neutrophils	$2\cdot5-7\cdot5 \times 10^9\,\text{l}^{-1}$
Lymphocytes	$1\cdot5-3\cdot5 \times 10^9\,\text{l}^{-1}$
Monocytes	$0\cdot2-0\cdot8 \times 10^9\,\text{l}^{-1}$
Eosinophils	$0\cdot04-0\cdot44 \times 10^9\,\text{l}^{-1}$
Basophils	$0\cdot015-0\cdot1 \times 10^9\,\text{l}^{-1}$

13.1.3 Coagulation parameters

Bleeding time	$<7\,\text{min}$
Clotting time (Lee White method)	$5-11\,\text{min}$
Partial thromboplastin time (PTT), activated	$25-60\,\text{s}$
Platelets	See Section 13.1.2 above
Prothrombin time (PT) (Quick, one-stage)	$12-16\,\text{s}$
International normalized ratio (INR)	$1\cdot0-1\cdot2$
Thrombin time (TT)	$\pm 5\,\text{s}$ of control

13.1.4 Blood gases and acid–base values

Base excess	$\pm 2 \cdot 3 \, \text{mmol} \, l^{-1}$
Bicarbonate, plasma	$21-30 \, \text{mmol} \, l^{-1}$
Bicarbonate, standard	$22-28 \, \text{mmol} \, l^{-1}$
Buffer base	$45-50 \, \text{mmol} \, l^{-1}$
$p\text{CO}_2$, arterial	$35-45 \, \text{mmHg}$
$p\text{CO}_2$, venous	$40-50 \, \text{mmHg}$
$p\text{O}_2$, arterial	<60 years: $>85 \, \text{mmHg}$
	$60-70$ years: $>75 \, \text{mmHg}$
	$70-80$ years: $60-70 \, \text{mmHg}$

13.1.5 Chemistry (alphabetical list)

(B), Whole blood; (P), plasma; (S), serum.

α-Amino acid nitrogen (P)	$30-55 \, \text{mg} \, l^{-1}$, $2 \cdot 1-4 \, \text{mmol} \, l^{-1}$
Aminolaevulinic acid (ALA)	See Section 13.7.5
Acid phosphatase (S), adults	$<11 \, \text{IU} \, l^{-1}$
Adrenocorticotrophic hormone (ACTH)	See Section 13.5
Aldosterone	See Section 13.5
Alkaline phosphatase (S), adults	$<100 \, \text{IU} \, l^{-1}$
Aminotransferases (S)	
AST (SGOT)	$<40 \, \text{IU} \, l^{-1}$
ALT (SGPT)	$<40 \, \text{IU} \, l^{-1}$
Ammonia nitrogen (B)	$400-800 \, \mu\text{g} \, l^{-1}$
Amylase (S)	$0 \cdot 8-1 \cdot 8$ Somogyi units ml^{-1}
	$3-10$ Wohlgemuth units ml^{-1}
	$86-268 \, \text{IU} \, l^{-1}$
Angiotensin converting enzyme	See Section 13.5
Ascorbic Acid (B)	$2-20 \, \text{mg} \, l^{-1}$, $11-113 \, \mu\text{mol} \, l^{-1}$
Bilirubin, total (S), adult	$<1 \cdot 3 \, \text{mg} \, dl^{-1}$, $<22 \, \mu\text{mol} \, l^{-1}$
	See also Section 13.7.1
Calcitonin	See Section 13.5
Biotin (S)	$20-100 \, \text{ng} \, dl^{-1}$, $0 \cdot 8-4 \cdot 1 \, \text{nmol} \, l^{-1}$
Carotenes	$25-150 \, \mu\text{g} \, dl^{-1}$ $0 \cdot 47-2 \cdot 78 \, \mu\text{mol} \, l^{-1}$
Calcium (S)	
Total	$85-105 \, \text{mg} \, l^{-1}$ $2 \cdot 1-2 \cdot 6 \, \text{mmol} \, l^{-1}$
Ionized	$40-50 \, \text{mg} \, l^{-1}$ $1 \cdot 0-1 \cdot 25 \, \text{mmol} \, l^{-1}$
Catecholamines (P)	See Section 13.5
Ceruloplasmin (S)	$20-46 \, \text{mg} \, dl^{-1}$, $13-30 \, \mu\text{mol} \, l^{-1}$
	See also Section 13.7.4

Chloride (P or S)	$3 \cdot 37 - 3 \cdot 72 \, g \, l^{-1}$, $95-105 \, mmol \, l^{-1}$
Cholesterol	See lipids
Chorionic gonadotropin	See Section 13.5
Cobalamin	See Section 13.6
Copper (P or S)	See Section 13.7.4
Coproporphyrin	See Section 13.7.5
Corticoids	See Section 13.5
Cortisol (P)	See Section 13.5
Creatine kinase (P or S)	See Section 13.7.3
Creatinine (S or P)	$6-15 \, mg \, l^{-1}$, $53-133 \, \mu mol \, l^{-1}$
Cyanocobalamin (S)	See Section 13.6
Estradiol and oestrogens	See Section 13.5
Fibrinogen (P)	$1 \cdot 5 - 4 \, g \, l^{-1}$
Folate (S)	See Section 13.6
Follicle-stimulating hormone	See Section 13.5
Gastrin (S or P)	See Section 13.5
Glucagon (P)	See Section 13.5
Glucose, fasting (P or S)	$0 \cdot 7 - 1 \cdot 1 \, g \, l^{-1}$, $3 \cdot 9 - 6 \cdot 1 \, mmol \, l^{-1}$
Growth hormone (S)	See Section 13.5
Haemoglobin (B)	Males: $13-18 \, g \, dl^{-1}$
	Females: $12-16 \, g \, dl^{-1}$
Homovanillic acid (HVA)	See Section 13.5
5-Hydroxy-indole acetic acid	See Section 13.5
Immunoglobulins (S)	(See also Section 13.7.2)
IgA	$<4 \, g \, l^{-1}$
IgD	$<50 \, mg \, l^{-1}$
IgE	$<1 \cdot 3 \, mg \, l^{-1}$
IgG	$<16 \, g \, l^{-1}$
IgM	$<2 \, g \, l^{-1}$
Insulin (S)	See Section 13.5
Iodine (S) (protein-bound, PBI)	$35-80 \, \mu g \, l^{-1}$, $276-630 \, nmol \, l^{-1}$
Iron (S)	See Section 13.7.4
Ketones (B)	$<30 \, mg \, l^{-1}$
17-Ketosteroids	See Section 13.5
Lactate (B)	
	Arterial: $30-70 \, mg \, l^{-1}$, $0 \cdot 3 - 0 \cdot 8 \, mmol \, l^{-1}$
	Venous: $50-200 \, mg \, l^{-1}$, $0 \cdot 56 - 2 \cdot 2 \, mmol \, l^{-1}$
Lipids (S)	
	Total: $4-10 \, g \, l^{-1}$
	Cholesterol: $1 \cdot 1 - 3 \cdot 0 \, g \, l^{-1}$,

	$2 \cdot 8 - 7 \cdot 8 \, \text{mmol} \, \text{l}^{-1}$
	Triglycerides: $0 \cdot 4 - 1 \cdot 5 \, \text{g} \, \text{l}^{-1}$
Luteinizing hormone (LH)	See Section 13.5
Magnesium (S)	$18 - 30 \, \text{mg} \, \text{l}^{-1}$, $0 \cdot 7 - 1 \cdot 2 \, \text{mmol} \, \text{l}^{-1}$
Nicotinic acid (S)	$1 \cdot 6 - 5 \cdot 0 \, \mu\text{g} \, \text{dl}^{-1}$, $130 - 410 \, \text{nmol} \, \text{l}^{-1}$
Pantothenic acid (B)	$20 - 190 \, \mu\text{g} \, \text{dl}^{-1}$, $0 \cdot 9 - 8 \cdot 7 \, \mu\text{mol} \, \text{l}^{-1}$
Phenylalanine (S)	$< 40 \, \text{mg} \, \text{l}^{-1}$, $< 242 \, \mu\text{mol} \, \text{l}^{-1}$
Phylloquinone (S)	$0 \cdot 9 - 7 \cdot 8 \, \mu\text{g} \, \text{dl}^{-1}$, $2 - 17 \, \text{nmol} \, \text{l}^{-1}$
Phosphatase (S)	
	Acid, adults: $< 4 \, \text{KA U dl}^{-1}$, $< 7 \, \text{IU} \, \text{l}^{-1}$
	Alkaline, adults: $< 13 \, \text{KA U dl}^{-1}$, $< 90 \, \text{IU} \, \text{l}^{-1}$
Phosphorus (P or S), inorganic	
	Adults: $2 \cdot 5 - 4 \cdot 5 \, \text{mg} \, \text{dl}^{-1}$, $0 \cdot 8 - 1 \cdot 5 \, \text{mmol} \, \text{l}^{-1}$
	Children: $4 \cdot 0 - 7 \cdot 0 \, \text{mg} \, \text{dl}^{-1}$, $1 \cdot 3 - 2 \cdot 3 \, \text{mmol} \, \text{l}^{-1}$
Porphobilinogen	See Section 13.7.5
Potassium (P)	$137 - 196 \, \text{mg} \, \text{l}^{-1}$, $3 \cdot 5 - 5 \, \text{mmol} \, \text{l}^{-1}$
Progesterone	See Section 13.5
Proteins (S)	
	Total: $6 \cdot 0 - 8 \cdot 4 \, \text{g} \, \text{dl}^{-1}$, $60 - 84 \, \text{g} \, \text{l}^{-1}$
	Albumin: $3 \cdot 0 - 5 \cdot 2 \, \text{g} \, \text{dl}^{-1}$, $30 - 52 \, \text{g} \, \text{l}^{-1}$
	Globulin: $2 \cdot 3 - 3 \cdot 7 \, \text{g} \, \text{dl}^{-1}$, $23 - 37 \, \text{g} \, \text{l}^{-1}$
	See also Sections 13.7.1 and 13.7.2
Protoporphyrin	See Section 13.7.5
Pyridoxine (S)	$30 - 80 \, \text{ng} \, \text{ml}^{-1}$
Pyruvate (B)	$3 - 10 \, \text{mg} \, \text{l}^{-1}$, $34 - 114 \, \mu\text{mol} \, \text{l}^{-1}$
Renin	See Section 13.5
Retinol	See Section 13.6
Riboflavin (S)	$4 - 24 \, \mu\text{g} \, \text{dl}^{-1}$, $100 - 640 \, \text{nmol} \, \text{l}^{-1}$
Serotonin	See 5-HIAA, Section 13.5
Sodium (P)	$3 \cdot 1 - 3 \cdot 4 \, \text{g} \, \text{l}^{-1}$, $135 - 148 \, \text{mmol} \, \text{l}^{-1}$
Sulphate, inorganic (S)	$9 - 60 \, \text{mg} \, \text{l}^{-1}$, $94 - 625 \, \mu\text{mol} \, \text{l}^{-1}$
Testosterone	See Section 13.5
Thiamine (S)	$2 \cdot 0 - 7 \cdot 5 \, \mu\text{g} \, \text{dl}^{-1}$, $75 - 280 \, \text{nmol} \, \text{l}^{-1}$
Thyroid-stimulating hormone (TSH)	See Section 13.5
Thyroxine (T4)	See Section 13.5

Thryoxine-binding globulin (TBG)	See Section 13.5
α-Tocopherol (P)	$5-20\,\mu g\,ml^{-1}$, $11\cdot6-46\cdot3\,\mu mol\,l^{-1}$
Transaminases	See aminotransferases
Triiodothyronine (T3)	See Section 13.5
Ubiquinone (S)	$40-115\,\mu g\,dl^{-1}$, $0\cdot46-1\cdot33\,\mu mol\,l^{-1}$
Urea nitrogen (B or S)	$80-250\,mg\,l^{-1}$, $5\cdot7-17\cdot9\,mmol\,l^{-1}$
Urea (B)	$171-535\,mg\,l^{-1}$, $2\cdot9-8\cdot9\,mmol\,l^{-1}$
Uric acid (S)	$15-70\,mg\,l^{-1}$, $89-417\,\mu mol\,l^{-1}$
Uroporphyrin	See Section 13.7.5
Vanillylmandelic acid (VMA)	See Section 13.5
Vitamin D (P)	$80-470\,ng\,dl^{-1}$, $2\cdot1-12\,nmol\,l^{-1}$
Zinc (S)	$0\cdot5-1\cdot5\,mg\,l^{-1}$, $8-23\,\mu mol\,l^{-1}$

13.2 Urinalysis

13.2.1 Physical values

Osmolality	$100-1000\,mOsm\,l^{-1}$ ($mmol\,kg^{-1}$)
pH	$4\cdot5-8\cdot0$ (average $=6\cdot0$)
Specific gravity	$1\cdot010-1\cdot025$
Volume, normal adult	$800-2000\,ml/24\,h$
Solids, total	$30-70\,g\,l^{-1}$
Microscopic examination	< 2 red or white cells per high-power field

13.2.2 Chemical values

α-Amino nitrogen	$50-300\,mg/24\,h$, $3\cdot6-21\cdot4\,mmol\,l/24\,h$
Aminolaevulinic acid (ALA)	$0\cdot1-7\cdot5\,mg/24\,h$, $0\cdot8-57\,\mu mol/24\,h$
Calcium	$100-300\,mg/24\,h$, $2\cdot5-7\cdot5\,mmol/24\,h$
Catecholamines	
Epinephrine	$< 20\,g/24\,h$, $< 109\,nmol/24\,h$
Norepinephrine	$< 100^{-1}\mu g/24\,h$, $< 591\,nmol/24\,h$
	See also Section 13.5
Chloride	$3\cdot55-8\cdot86\,g/24\,h$, $100-250\,mmol/24\,h$

Copper	15–45 μg/24 h, 0·25–0·75 μmol/24 h
Coproporphyrins	50–300 μg/24 h, 75–460 nmol/24 h
Isomers I : III ratio	1 : 4
Creatine, adults	< 250 mg/24 h, < 2 mmol/24 h
Creatinine	1–2 g/24 h, 8–18 mmol/24 h
Formiminoglutamic acid (FIGLU)	< 3 mg/24 h, < 17 μmol/24 h
After 15 g L-histidine	17 mg/24 h, 100 μmol/24 h
Homovanilic acid (HVA)	< 15 mg/24 h, < 82 μmol/24 h
Hydroxy-indole acetic acid (HIAA)	1–15 mg/24 h, 5–80 μmol/24 h
Magnesium	49–243 mg/24 h, 2–10 mmol/24 h
Nitrogen, total	5·4–21 g/24 h, 400–1500 mmol/24 h
Oxalate	15–40 mg/24 h, 167–444 μmol/24 h
Phosphate, inorganic	0·5–2·0 g/24 h, 16–65 mmol/24 h
Porphobilinogen	< 2 mg/24 h, < 9 μmol/24 h
Potassium	1·4–3·5 g/24 h, 35–90 mmol/24 h
Protein	< 100 mg/24 h
Sodium	1·8–12·9 g/24 h, 80–560 mmol/24 h
Urea	10–30 g/24 h, 167–500 mmol/24 h
Uric acid	0·2–0·6 g/24 h, 1·2–3·5 mmol/24 h
Urobilinogen	< 4 mg/24 h
Uroporphyrin	0–26 μg/24 h, 0–31 nmol/24 h

13.2.3 Clearance values (serum and urine)

Creatinine clearance (endogenous)	95–135 ml min^{-1}
Filtration fraction (FF)	17–23%
Glomerular filtration rate (GFR)	100–150 ml min^{-1}
Inulin	100–150 ml min^{-1}
p-Aminohippuric acid (PAH)	600–750 ml min^{-1}
Urea	Average standard: 40–65 ml min^{-1}
	Average maximum: 60–100 ml min^{-1}

13.3 Faecal analysis

13.3.1 Physical values

Mass	35–250 g/24 h
Water	60–80%

Osmolality	$284-430\,mOsm\,kg^{-1}$
Specific gravity	$1\cdot09$
pH	$7\cdot0-7\cdot5$
Microscopic examination	
Red blood cells	Absent
White blood cells	Few
Epithelial cells	Some
Crystals	Common (mainly oxalate, fatty acid and triple phosphate)
Fibres	Some undigested plant and dietary muscle fibres

13.3.2 Chemical values

Ammonia	$14-52\,mmol\,kg^{-1}$
Bicarbonate	$<30\,mmol\,kg^{-1}$
Bilirubin	$5-20\,mg/24\,h,\ 9-34\,\mu mol/24\,h$
Calcium	$7\cdot5-33\,mmol/24\,h$
Chloride	$18-106\,mg/24\,h,$ $0\cdot5-3\cdot0\,mmol/24\,h$
Coproporphyrin	$<50\,mg\,kg^{-1}\ (<76\,\mu mol\,kg^{-1})$ dry wt.
Fat (total lipid)	$<5\,g/24\,h,\ <30\%$ dry wt.
Iron	$5\cdot7-6\cdot7\,mg/24\,h,$ $100-120\,\mu mol/24\,h$
Nitrogen, total	$0\cdot5-2\cdot8\,g/24\,h,\ 64-200\,mmol/24\,h$
Organic acids, total	$100-400\,mmol\,kg$
Potassium	$0\cdot2-0\cdot6\,g/24\,h,\ 5-15\,mmol/24\,h$
Protoporphyrin	$<120\,mg\,kg^{-1}\ (<215\,\mu mol\,kg^{-1})$ dry wt.
Sodium	$10-110\,mg/24\,h,$ $0\cdot5-5\cdot0\,mmol/24\,h$
Trypsin	$60-650\,mg\,kg^{-1}$
Urobilinogen	$57-200\,mg/24\,h$
Uroporphyrin	$<60\,\mu g/24\,h,\ <75\,nmol/24\,h$

13.4 Cerebrospinal fluid

(Adult values)

pH	$7\cdot35-7\cdot40$

Osmolality	280–320 mOsm l^{-1} (mmol kg^{-1})
Total cell count	< 5 μl^{-1} (mononuclear cells)
Proteins, total	Lumbar: 150–450 mg l^{-1}
	Suboccipital: 140–360 mg l^{-1}
	Ventricular: 50–150 mg l^{-1}
Proteins, electrophoresis	
Albumin	56–76%
Prealbumin	2–7%
α_1-Globulin	2–8%
α_2-Globulin	3–12%
β-Globulin	4–14%
Gamma-globulin	3–13%
IgG	14–18 mg l^{-1}
IgA	2–3 mg l^{-1}
Transferrin	8–17 mg l^{-1}
α-Microglobulin	13–84 mg l^{-1}
α_1-Acid glycoprotein	2–4 mg l^{-1}
Nitrogen	Total: 11–16 mmol l^{-1}
	Non-protein: 8–14 mmol l^{-1}
	α-Amino: 0·66–1·05 mmol l^{-1}
Aminotransferases	20–50% of serum activity
Bicarbonate	22–25 mmol l^{-1}
Calcium	1·0–1·4 mmol l^{-1}
Chloride	120–130 mmol l^{-1}
Creatinine	57–93 μmol l^{-1}
Creatine kinase	< 10% of serum activity
Glucose	2·5–4·2 mmol l^{-1}
Lactate dehydrogenase	10–30% of serum activity
Potassium	2·6–3·3 mmol l^{-1}
Sodium	135–155 mmol l^{-1}
Urea	2·3–6·0 mmol l^{-1}

13.5 Hormones in blood and urine

Adrenocorticotropic hormone (ACTH), plasma	09.00 h: < 125 pg ml^{-1}
	24.00 h: < 35 pg ml^{-1}
Aldosterone	Serum (a.m.): 1–21 ng dl^{-1}
	Urine: 2–16 μg/24 h

Angiotensin-converting enzyme, serum	$18-67\,\mathrm{U\,ml^{-1}}$
Calcitonin, plasma (basal)	Males: $< 0\cdot155\,\mathrm{ng\,ml^{-1}}$
	Females: $< 0\cdot105\,\mathrm{ng\,ml^{-1}}$
Catecholamines (free), plasma	
Epinephrine	Supine: $< 110\,\mathrm{pg\,ml^{-1}}$
	Standing: $< 140\,\mathrm{pg\,ml^{-1}}$
Norepinephrine	Supine: $70-750\,\mathrm{pg\,ml^{-1}}$
	Standing: $200-1700\,\mathrm{pg\,ml^{-1}}$
Dopamine	$< 30\,\mathrm{pg\,ml^{-1}}$
Catecholamines, urine	
Epinephrine	< 2 years: $< 3\cdot5\,\mu\mathrm{g}/24\,\mathrm{h}$
	$2-10$ years: $< 10\,\mu\mathrm{g}/24\,\mathrm{h}$
	> 10 years: $< 20\,\mu\mathrm{g}/24\,\mathrm{h}$
Norepinephrine	< 2 years: $< 20\,\mu\mathrm{g}/24\,\mathrm{h}$
	$2-10$ years: $4-65\,\mu\mathrm{g}/24\,\mathrm{h}$
	> 10 years: $< 100\,\mu\mathrm{g}/24\,\mathrm{h}$
Dopamine	< 2 years: $< 140\,\mu\mathrm{g}/24\,\mathrm{h}$
	$2-4$ years: $40-260\,\mu\mathrm{g}/24\,\mathrm{h}$
	> 4 years: $65-400\,\mu\mathrm{g}/24\,\mathrm{h}$
Chorionic gonadotropins, beta subunit, serum	$< 5\,\mathrm{IU\,l^{-1}}$
	$< 9\,\mathrm{IU\,l^{-1}}$ (post-menopausal)
Corticoids, plasma	a.m.: $7-28\,\mu\mathrm{g\,dl^{-1}}$
	p.m.: $2-18\,\mu\mathrm{g\,dl^{-1}}$
Cortisol (free), urine	$24-108\,\mu\mathrm{g}/24\,\mathrm{h}$
Dopamine	See catecholamines
Estradiol, serum	Children: $< 1\,\mathrm{ng\,dl^{-1}}$
	Adult males: $1-5\,\mathrm{ng\,dl^{-1}}$
	Adult females:
	$3-40\,\mathrm{ng\,dl^{-1}}$ (pre-menopausal)
	$< 3\,\mathrm{ng\,dl^{-1}}$ (post-menopausal)
Estrogens, urine	Children: $< 10\,\mu\mathrm{g}/24\,\mathrm{h}$
	Adult males: $15-40\,\mu\mathrm{g}/24\,\mathrm{h}$
	Adult females:
	$15-80\,\mu\mathrm{g}/24\,\mathrm{h}$ (pre-menopausal)
	$< 20\,\mu\mathrm{g}/24\,\mathrm{h}$ (post-menopausal)
Follicle-stimulating hormone (FSH) serum	Children: $< 10\,\mathrm{IU\,l^{-1}}$
	Adult males: $< 20\,\mathrm{IU\,l^{-1}}$
	Adult females:
	$< 20\,\mathrm{IU\,l^{-1}}$ (non-midcycle)

	$< 40\,\mathrm{IU\,l^{-1}}$ (midcycle)
	$40{-}160\,\mathrm{IU\,l^{-1}}$ (post-menopausal)
Gastrin, serum	$< 300\,\mathrm{pg\,ml^{-1}}$
Glucagon, plasma	$0{\cdot}4{-}1{\cdot}4\,\mu\mathrm{g\,l^{-1}}$ ($115{-}402\,\mathrm{pmol\,l^{-1}}$)
Growth hormone, serum	Males: $< 5\,\mathrm{ng\,ml^{-1}}$
	Females: $< 10\,\mathrm{ng\,ml^{-1}}$
Homovanillic acid (HVA), urine	< 1 year:
	$< 35\,\mu\mathrm{g\,mg^{-1}}$ creatinine
	$1{-}2$ years:
	$< 23\,\mu\mathrm{g\,mg^{-1}}$ creatinine
	$2{-}14$ years:
	$< 13\,\mu\mathrm{g\,mg^{-1}}$ creatinine
	$14{-}18$ years:
	$< 2\,\mu\mathrm{g\,mg^{-1}}$ creatinine
	Adults: $< 8\,\mathrm{mg/24\,h}$
5-Hydroxyindole acetic acid (5-HIAA, serotonin), urine	$1{-}15\,\mathrm{mg/24\,h}$ ($5{-}80\,\mu\mathrm{mol/24\,h}$)
Insulin, serum	$< 25\,\mu\mathrm{U\,ml^{-1}}$
17-Ketosteroids, urine	< 10 years: $< 3\,\mathrm{mg/24\,h}$
	$10{-}14$ years: $2{-}7\,\mathrm{mg/24\,h}$
	Adult males: $6{-}21\,\mathrm{mg/24\,h}$
	Adult females: $4{-}17\,\mathrm{mg/24\,h}$
Luteinizing hormone (LH), serum	Children: $< 15\,\mathrm{IU\,l^{-1}}$
	Adult males: $< 24\,\mathrm{IU\,l^{-1}}$
	Adult females:
	$< 30\,\mathrm{IU\,l^{-1}}$ (non-midcycle)
	$30{-}150\,\mathrm{IU\,l^{-1}}$ (midcycle)
	$30{-}120\,\mathrm{IU\,l^{-1}}$ (post-menopausal)
Progesterone, serum	Males: $< 100\,\mathrm{ng\,dl^{-1}}$
	Pre-menopausal females:
	$< 70\,\mathrm{ng\,dl^{-1}}$ (follicular phase)
	$0{\cdot}2{-}2{\cdot}0\,\mu\mathrm{g\,dl^{-1}}$ (luteal phase)
Renin activity, plasma, Na-replete, upright	< 40 years: $0{\cdot}6{-}4{\cdot}3\,\mathrm{ng\,ml^{-1}\,h^{-1}}$
	> 40 years: $0{\cdot}6{-}3{\cdot}0\,\mathrm{ng\,ml^{-1}\,h^{-1}}$
Testosterone, serum	Males: total $300{-}1200\,\mathrm{ng\,dl^{-1}}$; free $9{-}30\,\mathrm{ng\,dl^{-1}}$
	Females: total $20{-}80\,\mathrm{ng\,dl^{-1}}$; free $0{\cdot}3{-}1{\cdot}9\,\mathrm{ng\,dl^{-1}}$
Thyroid-stimulating hormone (TSH), serum	$7\,\mathrm{mU\,l^{-1}}$

Thyroxine (T4), serum   Total: $50-135\,\mu g\,l^{-1}$
Free: $8-25\,\mu g\,l^{-1}$

Thyroxine-binding globulin
(TBG), serum $16-24\,mg\,l^{-1}$
Triiodothyronine (T3), serum, $0\cdot9-2\cdot3\,\mu g\,l^{-1}$
total
Vanillylmandelic acid (VMA),   < 1 year: $< 27\,\mu g\,mg^{-1}$ creatinine
urine   1–4 years: $< 18\,\mu g\,mg$ creatinine
4–10 years: $< 9\,\mu g\,mg^{-1}$ creatinine
10–18 years: $< 7\,\mu g\,mg^{-1}$ creatinine
Adults: $< 9\,\mu g\,mg^{-1}$ creatinine

13.6   Vitamins in blood (adult values)

Ascorbic acid (vitamin C), serum	$2-20\,mg\,l^{-1}$, $11-113\,\mu mol\,l^{-1}$
Biotin, serum	$20-100\,ng\,dl^{-1}$, $0\cdot8-4\cdot1\,nmol\,l^{-1}$
Carotenes, serum	$25-150\,\mu g\,dl^{-1}$, $0\cdot47-2\cdot78\,\mu mol\,l^{-1}$
Cobalamin (vitamin B_{12}), serum	$10-100\,ng\,dl^{-1}$, $150-750\,pmol\,l^{-1}$
B_{12}-binding capacity, serum	$0\cdot5-1\cdot8\,pg\,ml^{-1}$,
	$400-1300\,pmol\,l^{-1}$
Folate	
Serum	$1\cdot5-16\,ng\,ml^{-1}$, $3\cdot3-35\,nmol\,l^{-1}$
Red blood cells	$31-400\,ng\,ml^{-1}$, $67-800\,nmol\,l^{-1}$
Nicotinic acid, serum	$1\cdot6-5\cdot0\,\mu g\,dl^{-1}$, $130-410\,nmol\,l^{-1}$
Pantothenic acid, blood	$20-190\,\mu g\,dl^{-1}$, $0\cdot9-8\cdot7\,\mu mol\,l^{-1}$
Phylloquinone (vitamin K_1), serum	$0\cdot9-7\cdot8\,ng\,ml^{-1}$, $2-17\,nmol\,l^{-1}$
Pyridoxine (vitamin B_6), serum	$30-80\,ng\,ml^{-1}$
Retinol (vitamin A), serum	$20-100\,\mu g\,dl^{-1}$, $0\cdot75-3\cdot5\,\mu mol\,l^{-1}$
Retinol-binding protein, serum	$32-96\,mg\,l^{-1}$
Riboflavin (vitamin B_2), serum	$3\cdot8-24\,\mu g\,dl^{-1}$, $100-640\,nmol\,l^{-1}$
Thiamine (vitamin B_1), serum	$2\cdot0-7\cdot5\,\mu g\,dl^{-1}$, $75-280\,nmol\,l^{-1}$
α-Tocopherol (vitamin E), plasma	$5-20\,\mu g\,ml^{-1}$, $11\cdot6-46\cdot3\,\mu mol\,l^{-1}$
Ubiquinone, serum	$40-115\,\mu g\,dl^{-1}$, $0\cdot46-1\cdot33\,\mu mol\,l^{-1}$
Vitamin D, plasma	$80-470\,ng\,dl^{-1}$, $2\cdot1-12\,nmol\,l^{-1}$

13.7 Parameters of particular relevance to liver disease

13.7.1 Standard liver function tests

Total protein	$6 \cdot 0 - 8 \cdot 4 \, g \, dl^{-1}$, $60 - 84 \, g \, l^{-1}$
Albumin	$3 \cdot 0 - 5 \cdot 2 \, g \, dl^{-1}$, $30 - 52 \, g \, l^{-1}$
Globulin	$2 \cdot 3 - 3 \cdot 7 \, g \, dl^{-1}$, $23 - 37 \, g \, l^{-1}$
Bilirubin	< 1 month: $1 - 12 \, mg \, dl^{-1}$, $< 200 \, \mu mol \, l^{-1}$ (mainly indirect)
	1 month to adult, total: $< 1 \cdot 3 \, mg \, dl^{-1}$, $< 22 \, \mu mol \, l^{-1}$
	1 month to adult, direct: $< 0 \cdot 3 \, mg \, dl^{-1}$, $< 5 \, \mu mol \, l^{-1}$
Alkaline phosphatase (ALP)	< 10 years: up to $350 \, IU \, l^{-1}$
	10–15 years: up to $500 \, IU \, l^{-1}$
	Adults: $< 100 \, IU \, l^{-1}$
Aspartate aminotransferase (AST/SGOT)	$< 40 \, IU \, l^{-1}$
Alanine aminotransferase (ALT/SGPT)	$< 40 \, IU \, l^{-1}$
Prothrombin time (PT)	12–16 s
INR	$1 \cdot 0 - 1 \cdot 2$

13.7.2 Serum proteins

Protein electrophoresis	
Albumin	52–65% (of total)
Globulins	
$\alpha 1$	$2 \cdot 5 - 5 \cdot 0 \%$
$\alpha 2$	7–13%
β	8–14%
γ	12–22%
Prealbumin	$180 - 375 \, mg \, l^{-1}$
Immunoglobulins (g/l)	

	IgG	IgA	IgM
Neonates:	9–15	< 0·05	< 0·02
1–6 months:	3–6	< 0·5	< 0·6
6–12 months:	4–9	< 0·6	< 0·75

1–5 years:	5–11	< 1·5	< 1·0
5–12 years:	5–14	< 2·0	< 1·1
Adults:	6–16	< 4·0	< 2·0

α_1-Antitrypsin	$1-2\,\mathrm{g\,l^{-1}}$
Ceruloplasmin	See Section 13.7.4
Ferritin	See Section 13.7.4
Transferrin	See Section 13.7.4
Fibrinogen	$1\cdot5-4\cdot0\,\mathrm{g\,l^{-1}}$
Haptoglobin	$0\cdot6-2\cdot7\,\mathrm{g\,l^{-1}}$
α_1-Acid glycoprotein (orosomucoid)	$0\cdot38-1\cdot58\,\mathrm{g\,l^{-1}}$
Complement components	
C1 esterase inhibitor	$160-330\,\mathrm{mg\,l^{-1}}$
C3 (β1c globulin)	$0\cdot8-2\cdot0\,\mathrm{g\,l^{-1}}$
C4	$120-750\,\mathrm{mg\,l^{-1}}$
Total	41–90 haemolytic units

13.7.3 Serum enzymes

Aminotransferases	See Section 13.7.1
Alkaline phosphatase	See Section 13.7.1
Amylase	$< 300\,\mathrm{IU\,l^{-1}}$
Cholinesterase	$< 9\,\mathrm{IU\,l^{-1}}$
Creatine kinase (CPK)	$< 60\,\mathrm{IU\,l^{-1}}$
Lactate dehydrogenase (LDH)	Adults: $< 190\,\mathrm{IU\,l^{-1}}$
	Children: 2–5 times adult values
Leucine aminopeptidase (LA)	$< 50\,\mathrm{IU\,l^{-1}}$
5′-Nucleotidase	$< 10\,\mathrm{IU\,l^{-1}}$
Ornithine carbamoyl transferase (OCT)	$< 10\,\mathrm{IU\,l^{-1}}$

13.7.4 Iron and copper

Iron, serum	$55-170\,\mu\mathrm{g\,dl^{-1}}$, $10-30\,\mu\mathrm{mol\,l^{-1}}$
Total iron-binding capacity (TIBC)	$250-390\,\mu\mathrm{g\,dl^{-1}}$, $45-70\,\mu\mathrm{mol\,l^{-1}}$
Transferrin saturation	25–50%
Transferrin, serum	$1\cdot5-3\cdot4\,\mathrm{g\,l^{-1}}$
Ferritin, serum	Neonates: $< 200\,\mu\mathrm{g\,l^{-1}}$
	1 month: $200-600\,\mu\mathrm{g\,l^{-1}}$

	2–12 months: $< 200\,\mu g\,l^{-1}$
	1–15 years: $< 150\,\mu g\,l^{-1}$
	Adults: $< 200\,\mu g\,l^{-1}$
Copper, serum	Total: $60–180\,\mu g\,dl^{-1}$,
	$10–30\,\mu mol\,l^{-1}$
	Free: $< 12\,\mu g\,dl^{-1}$, $< 2\,\mu mol\,l^{-1}$
Copper, urinary	$15–45\,\mu g/24\,h$,
	$0\cdot25–0\cdot75\,\mu mol/24\,h$
Ceruloplasmin, serum	$20–46\,mg\,dl^{-1}$, $13–30\,\mu mol\,l^{-1}$
Copper, liver	$< 1\,\mu mol\,g$ dry wt.

13.7.5 Porphyrins

δ-Aminolevulinic acid (ALA)

Neonates

Plasma:
$< 75\,ng\,ml^{-1}$, $< 0\cdot57\,\mu mol\,l^{-1}$
Erythrocytes:
$370–1750\,ng\,ml^{-1}$, $2\cdot8–13\cdot3\,\mu mol\,l^{-1}$

Adults

Serum:
$< 100\,ng\,ml^{-1}$, $< 0.76\,\mu mol\,l^{-1}$
Erythrocytes:
$250–450\,ng\,ml^{-1}$, $1\cdot9–3\cdot4\,\mu mol\,l^{-1}$
Urine: See Section 13.2.2

Coproporphyrin

Neonates

Plasma:
$2–13\,ng\,ml^{-1}$, $3–20\,nmol\,l^{-1}$
Erythrocytes:
$10–70\,ng\,ml^{-1}$, $17–110\,nmol\,l^{-1}$

Adults

Plasma:
$4–15\,ng\,ml^{-1}$, $6–23\,nmol\,l^{-1}$
Erythrocytes:
$3–23\,ng\,ml^{-1}$, $5–35\,nmol\,l^{-1}$
Urine: See Section 13.2.2

Porphobilinogen

Neonates

Erythrocytes:
$230–700\,ng\,ml^{-1}$, $1–3\,\mu mol\,l^{-1}$

Adults

Serum:
$< 44\,ng\,ml^{-1}$, $< 190\,nmol\,l^{-1}$
Erythrocytes:
$150–400\,ng\,ml^{-1}$, $0\cdot7–1\cdot8\,\mu mol\,l^{-1}$
Urine: See Section 13.2.2

Protoporphyrin
  Neonates
    Plasma:
    $1-9\,\text{ng ml}^{-1}$, $1\cdot8-16\,\text{nmol l}^{-1}$
    Erythrocytes:
    $340-1350\,\text{ng ml}^{-1}$, $0\cdot6-$
      $2\cdot4\,\mu\text{mol l}^{-1}$

  Adults
    Serum: nil   nil
    Erythrocytes:
    $170-510\,\text{ng ml}^{-1}$, $0\cdot3-0\cdot9\,\mu\text{mol l}^{-1}$

Uroporphyrin
  Neonates
    Erythrocytes:
      $< 1\,\text{ng ml}^{-1}$, $< 1\cdot2\,\text{nmol l}^{-1}$

  Adults
    Serum: nil   nil
    Erythrocytes:
      $< 20\,\text{n ml}^{-1}$, $< 24\,\text{nmol l}^{-1}$
    Urine: See Section 13.2.2

Index

Anaemia (*continued*)
megaloblastic, 75–6, 221
nematode infections and, 267
pernicious, 14, 76
porphyrinuria in, 241
sickle-cell, 21, 227
sideroachrestic, 221
sideroblastic, 76, 227
sideropenic, 223
trematode infections and, 267
in Weil's disease, 261
Androgens, 142–4, 200
Angiosarcoma, 9
Anti-alcohol antibodies, 210, 215
Anti-ASPGP-R, *see* Autoantibodies
Anti-ENA, *see* Autoantibodies
Anti-HBcAg, *see* Hepatitis B serum
markers
Anti-HBeAg, *see* Hepatitis B serum
markers
Anti-HBsAg, *see* Hepatitis B serum
markers
Anti-LSP, *see* Autoantibodies
Anti-mitochondrial antibodies
(AMA), *see* Autoantibodies
Anti-nuclear antibodies (ANA), *see*
Autoantibodies
Antipyrine, 54
Anti-SLA, *see* Autoantibodies
Anti-smooth muscle antibodies
(SMA), *see* Autoantibodies
Antithrombin III, 68
Anti-thyroid antibodies, 124
α1-Antitrypsin, 31, 234–7
acute-phase reactant, 120, 236
deficiency, 110, 235–7, 248
neonatal hepatitis and, 247
phenotyping, 235–6
Aprindine, 199
Arboviruses, 96–7
Arenaviruses, 96–7
Argentinian haemorrhagic fever, 97
Aromatase, 143
Arthropathy, *see also* Rheumatoid
arthritis
in haemochromatosis, 226

Ascaris lumbricoides, 267
Ascites
bacterial peritonitis and, 62
differential diagnosis of, 61
in hepatic malignancy, 162
monitoring treatment of, 60
in tyrosinaemia, 244
pathogenesis of, 58–60
Ascorbic acid, *see* Vitamin C
Asialoglycoprotein receptor, 117
Asialotransferrin, *see* Transferrin
Aspartate aminotransferase (AST),
see also Aminotransferases
mitochondrial (mAST), 27, 214
pre-mAST, 27
Aspergillosis, 268
Aspirin, 193
Ataxiatelangiectasia syndrome, 168
Australia antigen, 85
Autoantibodies, serum, 112–18
anti-ASGP-R, 117, 127–9
anti-centromere, 112, 126
anti-DNA, 111, 113–14
anti-ENA, 114
anti-LSP, 117, 127–9
anti-mitochondrial (AMA), 115,
121, 124–6
sub-specificities of, 115
antinuclear (ANA), 112–14, 121,
124–5
sub-specificities of, 113
anti-SLA, 118, 127–9
anti-smooth muscle (SMA),
in alcoholic liver disease, 114,
125, 127, 207, 210, 215
in chronic active hepatitis, 110,
114, 124–6
drugs and, 195, 198, 202
in halothane hepatitis, 190
in haemochromatosis, 223
hepatocyte membrane antibodies
(HMA), 118, 127, 129
in Indian childhood cirrhosis, 233
liver autoantibodies, 127–9
liver-kidney microsomal (LKM)
antibodies, 116, 127–8

Renal failure (*continued*)
  in leptospirosis, 62, 264
  in paracetamol overdose, 193
  tetracyclines and, 195
  in tyrosinaemia, 245
  in viral infections, 62–3, 96
  in Wilson's disease, 232
Renal tubular acidosis
  in tyrosinaemia, 245
  in Wilson's disease, 232
Reverse T$_3$, *see* Triiodothyronine
Reye's syndrome, 152, 249, 252–3
Rheumatoid arthritis
  alkaline phosphatase in, 194–5
  antinuclear antibodies in, 113,
    124
  immune comlexes in, 118, 130
  ornithine carbamoyl transferase
    in, 194
Rheumatoid arthritis-associated
  antigen (RANA), 113, 132
Rheumatoid factor, 124
Rifampicin, 187, 196, 197
Rose–Bengal test, 40, 253
Rotor's syndrome, 45, 241, 249,
  250–1
Rubella, 96, 259

Salicylates, 194
Santa Marta hepatitis, 90
Sarcoidosis, 129, 258–60
Sarcoma, hepatic, 158
Schistosomiasis, 266–7
Sclerosing cholangitis, *see* Primary
  sclerosing cholangitis
Secondary iron overload, 221,
  226–7
Senecio alkaloids, 203
Septrin, 196
Seroconversion, 87
Serotonin, 174
Serum bile acids, *see* Bile acids
Serum globulins, *see* Globulins
Sex-hormone binding globulin
  (SHBG), 143

  in chronic liver disease, 144
Sex-hormones, 142–6
Sickle-cell anaemia
  haemolytic jaundice in, 21
  secondary iron overload in, 227
Sjogren's syndrome
  antinuclear antibodies in, 112,
    126
SLE, *see* Systemic lupus
  erythematosus
Sodium valproate, 193
Sodium balance, *see also*
  Hyponatraemia
  ascites and, 59, 60
  hepatorenal syndrome and, 63
Spherocytosis, congenital, 227
Spironolactone
  ascites and, 60
Spontaneous bacterial peritonitis,
  62
Stercobilin, 17
Stercobilinogen, 17
Streptococcus milleri, 261
Streptokinase, 67
Streptomycin, 197
Strongyloides stercoralis, 267
Sucrose haemolysis test, 73
Sulindac, 194
Sulphasalazine, 187, 195
Sulphonamides, 187, 195, 196
Sulphones, 197
Syphilis, 265
Systemic lupus erythematosus (SLE)
  antinuclear antibodies in,
    112–14, 126
  anti-mitochondrial antibodies in,
    115
  LE cells in, 111, 121
  immune complexes in, 118, 130
Taenia spp., 265
Tannic acid
  in haemagglutination tests, 136
  hepatotoxicity, 203
Technetium-diisopropylimino-
  diacetic acid
  cholescintigraphy, 246

Uric acid, blood
  in alcohol liver disease, 209, 215
  in glycogen storage diseases, 244
  in Wilson's disease, 232
Uric acid, urinary
  in Wilson's disease, 232
Urobilinogen, 13, 17, 20
Uroporphyrinogen decarboxylase,
  241
Ursodeoxycholate, 51

Varicella zoster, 96
Variegate porphyria, 239
Vasculitis
  immune complexes and, 130
Venereal diseases, 264–5
Venesection, see Phlebotomy
  therapy
Veno-occlusive disease, 203
Vinyl chloride, 203
Vitamins, fat-soluble
  bile salt metabolism and, 51
Vitamin B$_6$ deficiency
  sideroblastic anaemia and, 76
Vitamin B$_{12}$, 73
  alcohol and, 76, 211, 214
  hepatic abscesses and, 262
  idiopathic macrocytosis and, 75
  megaloblastic anaemia and, 76
  unsaturated, binding capacity
    in fibrolamellar carcinoma, 171
Vitamin C
  iron stores and, 225
Vitamin D
  calcium metabolism and, 152–3

Vitamin K
  coagulopathy and, 33, 70, 72,
    171
  in haemostasis, 69

Warfarin
  induction of gammaglutamyl
    transpeptidase, 29
  prothrombin time and, 70
Warts, plantar
  autoantibodies and, 124
Watson–Schwartz test, 239
White blood cells
  function of, 78
Wilson's disease, 227–32
  asymptomatic, screening for,
    232–3
  autoantibodies in, 125, 127–9
  diagnostic tests for, 229–31
  in differential diagnosis, 110,
    216, 251
  haemolytic jaundice in, 29, 232
  monitoring therapy in, 232
Weil's disease, 263–4

Xenelamine, 197

Yellow fever, 96

Zieve's syndrome, 21, 77